HARLEY-DAVIDSON

TRIVIA BOOK

Uncover The History & Facts Every Fan
Needs To Know!

By

Matt Hoffman

Bridge Press
support@bridgepress.org

Please consider writing a review!
Just visit: purplelink.org/review

ISBN: 978-1-955149-21-1

Acknowledgements:
Thank you to the community of riders who ride with
passion!

TABLE OF CONTENTS

Introduction 1

Chapter 1:
The Early History and Founders of the
Harley-Davidson Motor Company 3

Trivia Time!... 3

Answer Key:.. 9

Facts, Factoids, and Interesting Stories 10

Chapter 2:
World War I and the Roaring Twenties 15

Trivia Time... 15

Answer Key.. 20

Facts, Factoids, and Interesting Stories 22

Chapter 3:
The Great Depression, the 1930s, and
the Second World War 27

Trivia Time... 27

Answer Key.. 33

Facts, Factoids, and Interesting Stories 35

Chapter 4:

Post-World War II, the Korean War, and the Motorcycles of the '50s and '60s ... 40

Trivia Time 40

Answer Key 46

Facts, Factoids, and Interesting Stories 47

Chapter 5:
The Vietnam War Era and the AMF Years (1960s–80s) 51

Trivia Time 51

Answer Key 57

Facts, Factoids, and Interesting Stories 59

Chapter 6:
After the AMF and the 1990s 62

Trivia Time 62

Answer Key 68

Facts, Factoids, and Interesting Stories 69

Chapter 7:
The End of the '90s, Into the Aughts 72

Trivia Time 72

Answer Key 77

Facts, Factoids, and Interesting Stories 79

Chapter 8:

2010s to the Present...................... 81

Trivia Time............................ 81

Answer Key............................ 87

Facts, Factoids, and Interesting Stories 88

Chapter 9:
Harley-Davidson in Stunts, Films,
Television, and the Media.................... 91

Trivia Time............................ 91

Answer Key............................ 97

Facts, Factoids, and Interesting Stories 98

Chapter 10:
Motorcycle Clubs, Criminal Motorcycle
Gangs, and the Harley-Davidson 102

Trivia Time............................ 102

Answer Key............................ 108

Facts, Factoids, and Interesting Stories 110

Chapter 11:
The History of Harley-Davidson in the
Racing Circuit 113

Trivia Time............................ 113

Answer Key............................ 119

Facts, Factoids, and Interesting Stories 120

Chapter 12:
Harley-Davidson, the Motorcycle, and Timeless Rock Music 122

Trivia Time 122

Answer Key 128

Facts, Factoids, and Interesting Stories...........130

Chapter 13:
Celebrity Harley-Davidson Owners ... 132

Trivia Time 132

Answer Key 139

Facts, Factoids, and Interesting Stories...........140

Chapter 14:
Accessories, Gear, and Parts.............. 144

Trivia Time 144

Answer Key 150

Facts, Factoids, and Interesting Stories...........151

Chapter 15:
Superstition, Misconceptions, and Myths of Motorcycles and Harley-Davidsons 152

Trivia Time 152

Answer Key 158

Facts, Factoids, and Interesting Stories...........160

Conclusion.. **163**

INTRODUCTION

Harley-Davidson motorcycles are among the most iconic motorbikes in the world, made both renowned and notorious through the brand's connection to the U.S. military, nomadic travelers, competitive racers, and criminal gangs. Their sleek design, powerful engines, and rich history have captured the imaginations of men and women across the globe. In many ways, the company of Harley-Davidson established the prominent motorcycle culture best remembered through movies and television shows such as *Terminator 2*, *Rocky III*, *Pulp Fiction*, *Mayans M.C.*, *Ghost Rider*, *Hell Ride*, *Easy Rider*, *Sons of Anarchy*, and *The Wild One*.

The Harley-Davidson Motor Company was born for a love of the road, the pursuit of adventure, and the desire for innovation. The bikes and culture that arose were birthed from the minds of Arthur Davidson, Walter Davidson, William Davidson, and William Harley, whose work would become a staple and dynamic component of American society. This book will cover trivia about the motorcycles, racers, inventors, and different facets of the history of the Harley-Davidson

Motor Company from its inception in 1903 to the outlook for the business from 2021 onward.

The chapters will be formatted with a twenty-question trivia quiz focusing on the topic of the section, an answer key, and a "Did You Know" section. Regardless of whether you are a massive Harley-Davidson enthusiast or a casual motorcycle fan, this book can help you learn more about the bikes, individuals, and events that define the Harley-Davidson Motor Company's incredibly fascinating history and test your knowledge of one of the most famous motorbikes in the world.

Now, on to the fun part to see how well you know the history of the incomparable Harley-Davidson.

CHAPTER 1:

THE EARLY HISTORY AND FOUNDERS OF THE HARLEY-DAVIDSON MOTOR COMPANY

TRIVIA TIME!

1. In an act that would inspire William S. Harley and Arthur Davidson, which term did inventor and charlatan Edward J. Pennington coin in 1895?
   a. Motorbike
   b. Motorcycle
   c. Motorized scooter
   d. Bicycle

2. Which company revolutionized the lightweight internal combustion engine at the end of the 19th century (and would play a major role in the development of Harley-Davidson)?
   a. Cannstatt-Daimer
   b. Peugeot
   c. Dion-Bouton

d. Excelsior

3. Which city was home to the founders of the Harley-Davidson Motor Company?

   a. Milwaukee, Wisconsin
   b. Chicago, Illinois
   c. Ann Arbor, Michigan
   d. St. Louis, Missouri

4. Who did William S. Harley work with to help develop a powerful motorized engine to improve his original 1901 prototype?

   a. C. H. Lang
   b. Walter Davidson
   c. Gottlieb Daimler
   d. Ole Evinrude

5. Which friend of Arthur Davidson worked with him and William Harley on their design?

   a. Nicholas-Joseph Cugnot
   b. George Baldwin
   c. Henry Melk
   d. Henry Ford

6. In which year was the Harley-Davidson Motor Company founded?

   a. 1898
   b. 1903
   c. 1905
   d. 1910

7. In 1904, Henry Meyer became the first person to have bought a motorcycle from Harley-Davidson. Who was the first entrepreneur to begin selling them in 1905?

    a. Charles H. Lang in Chicago
    b. Thomas Edison in West Orange
    c. Ole Evinrude in Milwaukee
    d. Henry Ford in Detroit

8. What was the name of the first catalog magazine published by the Harley-Davidson Motor Company in 1906?

    a. *The Kings of the Road*
    b. *Riders of the Storm*
    c. *Chestnut Street Motorbikes*
    d. *Silent Gray Fellows*

9. Chestnut Street (now Juneau Avenue) was home to the first two Harley-Davidson production houses (as a shed and then as a factory).

    a. True
    b. False

10. At the Seventh Annual Federation of American Motorcyclists Endurance and Reliability Contest in 1908, Walter Davidson scored a perfect 1,000 points.

    a. True
    b. False

11. Harley-Davidson motorcycles were the first motorbikes to include a clutch.

    a. True
    b. False

12. Which was the first police force to buy Harley-Davidson for their department in 1908?

    a. Milwaukee Police
    b. Detroit Police
    c. Indianapolis Police
    d. St. Paul Police

13. The famous logo of Harley-Davidson is called:

    a. "Sword and Shield"
    b. "Stripe and Targe"
    c. "Bar and Shield"
    d. "Blade and Buckler"

14. Which type of new engine, introduced in 1909, would go on to revolutionize motorcycles?

    a. V-twin
    b. Flat Twin
    c. V-4
    d. Inline

15. At the start of the 1910s, which company was the greatest competition for Harley-Davidson in the racing circuit?

    a. Triumph
    b. Royal Enfield

c. Peugeot

d. Indian

16. To which country did the Harley-Davidson Motor Company begin exporting motorcycles and products in the year 1912?

a. Imperial Russia

b. Brazil

c. Egypt

d. Imperial Japan

17. In which year did Harley-Davidson start their Racing Department?

a. 1910

b. 1912

c. 1913

d. 1915

18. Sidecars were first introduced to Harley-Davidson bikes in 1910.

a. True

b. False

19. Which magazine did Harley-Davidson publish for the first time in 1916?

a. *Planes, Trains, and Automobiles*

b. *The Motorcycle Aficionado*

c. *The Enthusiast*

d. *Harley-Davidson Publications*

20. The fundamental construction of the Harley-Davidson has changed dramatically over the past 118 years and is almost unrecognizable from its original design.

   a. True
   b. False

ANSWER KEY:

1. B: Motorcycle

2. C: Dion-Bouton

3. A: Milwaukee, Wisconsin

4. C: Arthur Davidson

5. C: Henry Melk

6. B: 1903

7. A: Charles H. Lang in Chicago

8. D: *Silent Gray Fellows*

9. True

10. True

11. True

12. B: Detroit Police Department

13. C: "Bar and Shield"

14. A: V-twin

15. D: Indian

16. D: Japan

17. C: 1913

18. False

19. C: *The Enthusiast*

20. False

FACTS, FACTOIDS, AND INTERESTING STORIES

- Air-cooled single-cylinder engines, based on the Count De Dion Company's prototype, were first imported into the United States from France in 1896.

  - They were taken apart, rebuilt, and modified by American mechanics to become the standard for most motorbike engines during the early years of motorcycle production.

- The first Indian motorcycle was built in 1902 by George Hendee and Oscar Hedström.

- In 1902, a year before the Harley-Davidson Motor Company was founded, there were at least thirteen motorcycle factories in the United States.

  - All were using a variation of the De Dion archetype and were the inspiration for the production of Harley-Davidson engines in the coming year.

- Silent pipes were dangerous for motorcyclists.

  - Loud pipes saved bikers' lives.

- William Harley was a draftsman, and Arthur Davidson worked as a pattern maker at the same manufacturing company in Milwaukee prior to working together as hobby engineers.

- Milwaukee was the perfect place for experimentation with transportation, as the city was packed with different forms of travel, including horse-drawn carriages, bicycles, and electric streetcars.

  o This allowed for Harley and the Davidsons to begin experimenting with their designs and early models of motorcycles.

- 1903 is one of the most important years of vehicular innovation in the United States, filled with incredible ingenuity and initiative.

  o In Milwaukee, Wisconsin, the Davidson brothers, and Harley were building their first motorcycles.

  o In Kitty Hawk, North Carolina, Wilbur and Orville Wright built their first aircraft, the Wright Flyer.

  o In Dearborn, Michigan, Henry Ford was working on the Model A car.

- In 1907, Walter Davison rode a prototype of the twin in an endurance race that was to run from Chicago, Illinois, to Kokomo, Indiana. He scored a perfect 1,000 points.

  o Only two other racers scored and kept 1,000 points.

- Harley-Davidson motorcycles were mistakenly given a different name in the *New York Times*.

- In 1908, Harley-Davidson motorcycles became recognized on the east coast following Walter Davidson's victory at the National Endurance Contest.
  - With this win, he scored a perfect 1,000 points.
  - He rode through the New York state Catskill Mountains and beat out sixty-five other riders who were riding on seventeen various types of motorcycles.
  - This included the increasingly popular Indian motorcycles.
- The *New York Times* wrote of the victory, identifying the bike as a "Howard Davidson."
- The 1909 advertisements that marketed Harley-Davidson motorcycles promoted the company's exceptional build quality under the phrase "Built on Honor."
- V-twin engines were developed in 1889 by Gottlieb Daimler.
  - Harley-Davidson introduced its first V-twin engine in 1909.
    - It was difficult to drive because of the lack of a clutch.
      - The V-twin engine would be reintroduced in 1912 when a rotating grip

accelerator and a clutch were installed on the motorcycle.

- This was a year after the Indian motorcycle introduced the V-twin to their motorcycles.
- These engines had a leather strap or chain for the transmission.

- A stock racer from Harley-Davidson in 1910 cost $275 (inflation puts it at about $7,667).
- The earliest formation of motorcycle clubs started around 1911 in Milwaukee.

  o One example was the Cream City Motorcycle Club, which was founded by Milwaukee Harley dealer Bill Knuth.

    - They formed events such as the Knuth's Kollege, Midnight Mystery Tour, and the Badger Derby.

- From 1911, there have been legends of Harley-Davidsons being buried all around Milwaukee, including in landfills and city dumps, as well as in Lake Michigan.

  o These bikes may be lying beneath factories, apartment buildings, and other locations around the city because of their manner of disposal in the 1910s.

- The Parts and Accessories Department was formed in 1912.

- William Harley was put in charge of the racing department.
- In 1914, the kick-start, two-speed clutches, and footboards were three innovations that revolutionized motorcycle production.
- Harley-Davidson Motor Company's sidecars were first introduced in 1914.
- The Wrecking Crew made its debut in Venice in the year 1915.
- Electric lights, better lubrication, and the three-speed hand-shift transmission furthered the improvement of motorcycles in 1915.

  o Harley-Davidson notably won the famed 1916 Dodge City 300 thanks to their trained pit crews with support capabilities.

CHAPTER 2:

WORLD WAR I AND THE ROARING TWENTIES

TRIVIA TIME

1. The Mexican Revolutionary and legendary rebel Francisco "Pancho" Villa was pursued along the Mexican border by American soldiers on Harley-Davidson motorcycles with machine gun-armed sidecars with modified armor plates.

    a. True
    b. False

2. How much of the company was changed to be exclusively dedicated to the war effort during WWI?

    a. ½
    b. ¼
    c. ⅛
    d. ⅓

3. What color were Harley-Davidson motorcycles painted for the military during WWI?

    a. Navy blue
    b. Army green

c. Jet black

d. Beige tan

4. Special sidecars were designed to be outfitted with machine guns in Europe and in America for both combat and border patrols.

    a. True

    b. False

5. The bicycle industry nearly went bankrupt during the years the United States was involved in WWI.

    a. True

    b. False

6. What happened to civilian motorcycle production in Britain during WWI?

    a. Production of civilian motorcycles was extremely prosperous.

    b. British businesses went bankrupt as a result of the war.

    c. British motorcycle companies shut down all non-military bike production and focused on the war effort.

    d. American motorcycle corporations bought all the civilian motorcycles.

7. Which part of motorcycle culture came to a halt across the U.S. because of the war?

    a. Cross-country driving

    b. Motorcycle jousting

c. Stunt driving

d. Racing

8. What was the name of the training school that Harley-Davidson started in 1917 to train military mechanics to work on Harley-Davidsons?

    a. The Harley-Davidson Mechanics School

    b. The Quartermasters School

    c. The Motorcycle Academy of the United States

    d. The Military Mechanical Campus

9. What did the training school become after WWI?

    a. The American Motorcycle School

    b. The Mechanics University

    c. The Motorcycle Maintenance College

    d. Harley-Davidson Service School

10. The first American to enter the German Empire at the end of the First World War rode into the country on a Harley in 1918.

    a. True

    b. False

11. How big was the Big Twin engine in 1921?

    a. 56 cubic inches

    b. 74 cubic inches

    c. 64 cubic inches

    d. 80 cubic inches

12. What caused Harley-Davidson Motor Company to suffer its first major financial loss in 1921?

a. An economic recession
b. Fire damage to the building slowed production
c. A worker stealing a patent for one of the engines, requiring the company to go to court
d. Shutting down the factory for a month due to a remodeling project

13. Which type of motorized vehicle contributed to the financial losses of the Harley-Davidson Motor Company?

    a. Speedboats
    b. Aircrafts
    c. Automobiles
    d. Mopeds

14. Which Harley-Davidson model was the top seller in 1924?

    a. Model 12
    b. Model B
    c. Model 66
    d. Model JE

15. In which year did Harley-Davidson take out a patent on a shaft-drive system?

    a. 1920
    b. 1922
    c. 1925
    d. 1929

16. Which design feature was introduced for the first time on the 1925 Harley-Davidson Model JD?

a. Vertical battery
b. New steering system
c. New tire structure
d. Aligned foot brake arrangement

17. Which motorcycle club did Bill Knuth found in Milwaukee that became one of the first local MCs in the city?

    a. The Milwaukee Motorcycle Club
    b. The Cream City Motorcycle Club
    c. Knuth's Motorcycle Club
    d. The Harley-Davidson Motorcycle Club

18. In 1929, at the start of the Great Depression, which famous engine did Harley-Davidson introduce?

    a. 21-cubic-inch single engine
    b. 45-cubic-inch V-twin flathead
    c. 74-cubic-inch Big Twin engine
    d. 35-cubic-inch flat-twin sport

19. Which company won a lawsuit against Harley-Davidson in 1929?

    a. Indian
    b. Triumph
    c. Eclipse
    d. Ford

20. William S. Harley was happy with the outcome of the lawsuit in 1929.

    a. True
    b. False

ANSWER KEY

1. True

2. D: ⅓.

3. B: Army green

4. True

5. False

6. C: The British shut down all non-military bike production and focused on the war effort.

7. D: Racing

8. B: Quartermaster's School

9. D: Harley-Davidson Service School

10. True

11. B: 74-cubic-inch Big Twin engine

12. A: An economic recession

13. C: Automobile

14. D: Model JE

15. C: 1925

16. A: Vertical battery

17. B: Cream City Motorcycle Club

18. D: F-Head V-twin

19. C: Eclipse

20. False

FACTS, FACTOIDS, AND INTERESTING STORIES

- Side-valve engines were developed during WWI and became the standard engine during the late 1910s.
- Corporal Roy Holtz of Chippewa Falls, Wisconsin, was the first American soldier to enter the German Empire and did so riding on a Harley-Davidson motorcycle, which was also equipped with a sidecar.
- For racing, the overhead valve and overhead cam motorcycles were heavily favored, but converting these sport motorcycles to everyday use proved to be an infuriating frustration for mechanics and riders.
  - Motors had to be disassembled and cleaned out every time to protect them.
- Pancho Villa rode a 1914 Hendee Special, although he is best remembered riding atop a horse while leading his guerrilla forces in Mexico.
- After WWI, Harley-Davidson was kept afloat by the foreign market for American motorcycles but domestically struggled as few returning customers repeated purchases from the company.
  - Future American-made Harley-Davidson models now also had to compete with automobiles as

well as the cheaper, lighter British models that became popular in the early 1920s.

- Harley-Davidson famously has an unsolved mystery surrounding the 1911 portion of the factory on Juneau Avenue.

  o In the 1920s, test rider and factory racer Albert "Squibb" Henrich was told by Edwin "Sherbie" Becker of a hidden room where old belt-drive motorcycles were walled up behind a gigantic concrete wall near the elevator in the cellar.

    ▪ The legend of the motorcycle graveyard in the walls of factories and buildings in and around Milwaukee (as well as in dumps along Lake Michigan) became commonplace throughout the 20th century.

- The Cream City Motorcycle Club was responsible for uniting fans of the Harley- Davidson motorcycle in Milwaukee. It organized meetups to enjoy one another's company, eat together, discuss riding, teach mechanics, share advice, and deliberate the history of Harley-Davidson.

  o This club had been around since 1911.

- During WWI, Harley-Davidson motorcycles proved their reliability and power as they were able to maneuver comfortably through the French mud on the front.

- o William H. Davidson is quoted saying, "Harley got its deepest breath over in the mud in France."
- After the First World War, Harley-Davidson actively altered its selling practices to help boost sales to accommodate a return to the civilian market.
  - o In the United States, there were several drops in sales after the war.
  - o Walter Davidson stated in 1911, "The day of selling motorcycles sitting in your store, waiting for the customer to come to you has gone by."
  - o Returning to selling motorcycles and accessories on the civilian level had to change to focus on recovering from the war.
- Leslie "Red" Parkhurst rode a Harley-Davidson 61-cubic-inch racing bike which, in 1920, broke twenty-three speed records.
- The Sport model motorcycle was introduced by the Harley-Davidson Motor Company in 1919.
  - o It featured a 584cc engine, which was twice the size of the standard engine of the Indian light twin at the time.
  - o It was a middleweight bike that was "not a lightweight," as it was advertised in the catalogs featuring motorcycles for sale.
  - o It was the first flathead introduced by the company.
  - o It was rather expensive.

- It cost $445, which is equivalent to about $9,000 today.
- It was cheaper to buy a previously owned Model T Ford than a Sport.
- The model fell out of favor by the start of 1924.

- Flatheads became popular during the 1920s and were viewed as the standard Harley-Davidson for many riders through the 1920s into the 1940s.
- The minimal design of the Sport model had a magneto ignition but did not have lights on the front of the vehicle.
- The Banjo Two Cam was introduced in 1923 with eight valves and a double overhead cam.
- Hill climbing became the most popular sport on motorcycles during the 1930s, and Harley-Davidsons were a favorite ride.
- The first teardrop gas tank was added to the Harley JD model in 1925, and it later became the standard for Harley-Davidson motorcycles.
- Harley-Davidson reintroduced the single-cylinder motorcycle, which had not been produced since 1918.

  o The Models A, AA, B, and BA had both the overhead-valve and side-valve engine configurations.

- The JDH Two Cam was introduced in 1927.

- o This bike was a road variety of the competition motorcycle.
  - ▪ It was originally created by Bill Ottaway in 1919.
- In 1928, the two-cam engine was added to all the JD series.
- A V-twin 750, the Flathead 45, was introduced in 1929 and included the twirl principle from Harry Ricardo's design.
  - o It remained in use until 1972.
- Harley-Davidson was sued and forced to pay $1.1 million to the Eclipse Company for infringement of a patent for a clutch system.
  - o Walter Davidson was shocked by the loss and the amount Harley-Davidson was forced to pay and may have never gotten over it.

CHAPTER 3:

THE GREAT DEPRESSION, THE 1930S, AND THE SECOND WORLD WAR

TRIVIA TIME

1. What was the minimum price of a basic Sport model Harley-Davidson between 1926 and 1930?

   a. $150
   b. $330
   c. $250
   d. $210

2. During the Great Depression, an increase in which type of taxes heavily impacted sales of Harley-Davidsons in the southern hemisphere?

   a. Commonwealth tariffs
   b. Federal income taxes
   c. Social security taxes
   d. Import tariffs on rubber

3. What was the standard outfit of a Harley-Davidson rider in the 1930s?

a. Bicycle helmet, sneakers, T-shirts, and shorts
b. Coat, fedora, glasses, and gloves
c. Suit jacket, button-downs, dress shoes, trousers
d. Leather jackets, fly helmets, tall boots, and goggles

4. Which of the following did Harley-Davidson debut in 1930?

    a. 250cc flat head single cylinder
    b. 600cc Scout V-twin cylinder
    c. 500cc flathead single cylinder
    d. 585cc Sport

5. The Twin engines were considered "cool," while the single-engine was thought to be "dorky."

    a. True
    b. False

6. What was an advantage of the new flathead Seventy-Four (Model V) over the F-head V-twins?

    a. Prettier and brassier
    b. Lighter and faster
    c. Longer and wider
    d. More powerful and agile

7. What was the most famous motorcycle Harley-Davidson introduced in the 1930s?

    a. Chief
    b. Sportster
    c. Knucklehead

d. Café Racer

8. What became a defining feature of the "California" look designed by Tom Sifton?

   a. Oval tail lights
   b. Saddlebags
   c. Chrome-plated high-rise handlebars
   d. Rounded gas tank

9. Which Harley model was introduced for the first time in 1937?

   a. BX series
   b. MA series
   c. FL series
   d. WL series

10. In 1940, which race did Babe Tancrede win on his WLDR model Harley-Davidson?

    a. Daytona 200
    b. Black Hills Rally
    c. Daytona 500
    d. Catskill Races

11. In which year did the Knucklehead become the most popular selling motorcycle in the United States?

    a. 1939
    b. 1940
    c. 1941
    d. 1942

12. The Quartermaster School did not restart when the Americans entered World War II, and Harley-

Davidson stopped producing motorcycles during the war.

    a. True

    b. False

13. Which award was given to the Harley-Davidson Motor Company for their production of motorcycles?

    a. Medal of Honor

    b. Naval Cross

    c. Distinguished Service Medal

    d. Army-Navy "E" Award

14. How many Harleys are estimated[1] to have been used in the Second World War?

    a. 50,000

    b. 70,000

    c. 80,000

    d. 100,000

15. Which Harley-Davidson founders died during WWII?

    a. Walter Davidson and William S. Harley

    b. William Davidson and Arthur Davidson

    c. William S. Harley and Arthur Davidson

    d. None

---

[1] Please note there are varying numbers regarding how much of Harley-Davidson Motor Company was dedicated to the cause, I am looking for the official estimation.

16. Which Harley-Davidson motorcycle series was introduced in 1941?

    a. FL series
    b. RX series
    c. DC series
    d. AC series

17. Which military role did Harley-Davidsons play during WWII?

    a. Carrying weapons
    b. Reconnaissance
    c. Transport of prisoners
    d. Logistics support

18. What were the top two models sold to the military during the Second World War for American troops?

    a. VLD and Model D
    b. WLA and XA
    c. Forty-Five and Model V
    d. VLH and UL

19. Which accessory added to the maneuverability of the WLA model to permit more flexibility for the rider than ever before?

    a. Sidecars
    b. Machine guns
    c. A third wheel
    d. Saddlebags

20. Military Police (MP) had no use for the Harley-Davidson motorcycles during the war.

a. True
b. False

ANSWER KEY

1. D: $210

2. A: Commonwealth tariffs

3. D: Leather jackets, fly helmets, tall boots, and goggles

4. C: 500cc (30.5-cubic-inch) flathead single

5. True

6. B: Faster and lighter

7. C: Knucklehead

8. C: Chrome-plated high-rise handlebars

9. D: WL series

10. A: Daytona 200

11. C: 1941

12. False

13. D: Army-Navy "E" Award

14. C: 80,000

15. A: Walter Davidson and William S. Harley

16. A: FL Series

17. B: Reconnaissance

18. B: WLA and XA

19. D: Saddlebags

20. False

FACTS, FACTOIDS, AND INTERESTING STORIES

- The cheap-to-build VL models did not sell well in the 1930s due to the Depression.
- The first Sixty-One show model quietly sold for the first time in January 1936.

  o Butch Quirk famously rode a sidecar-equipped Sixty-One model in a 350-mile endurance race for the Portland Oregon Rose City Motorcycle Club in early February of that year.

  o It quickly became popularized during the first couple of months due to victories at local racetracks and unofficial competitions.

    ▪ Became a massively popular model.

- The XA model of Harley-Davidson motorcycles was based on parts and blueprints taken off a captured German BMW R71 from the Bavarian Motor Works and other German motorcycles from WWII.
- Because the Harley-Davidson motorcycle was frequently the first vehicle to be seen in the cities, villages, and towns freed from Nazi occupation across the European continent by the Allied forces, especially by the American services, the motorcycles were given the moniker "Liberators."
- Three of the four original Harley-Davidson founders died in this era:

- William A. Davidson died in 1937 at 67.
- Walter Davidson passed in 1942 at 66 years of age.
- William S. Harley followed his co-founders to the grave the subsequent year in 1943 at the age of 63.

- The Harley-Davidson Motor Company received a total of four Army-Navy "E" Awards for service in the Second World War.
- Harley-Davidson was the principal exporter and supplier of motorcycles to the Allied War effort.
- Imperial Japan produced Harley-Davidsons in the 1930s when they had a licensing deal with the Japanese company Rikuo.
  - Rikuo produced about 18,000 motorcycles.
- Servi-car premiered in 1932 and ran in production until 1973.
- The motorcycles that were built for the military were made to be adaptable and strong. They could travel comfortably and reliably through a variety of different terrains, including paved highways, cobblestone streets, forest paths, dirt roads, jungle terrain, sand dunes, and mountain trails alike.
- The overhead-valve 61-cubic-inch (1000cc) Knucklehead debuted in 1936.
- Motorcycles were an excellent vehicle for transport, carrying goods and materials.

- The 1938 Harley-Davidson Model U was used for commercial purposes and could carry multiple packages, gear, equipment, and a spare tire.
- Like the World War I production of motorcycles, Harley-Davidson nearly stopped all production of civilian bikes during the period of American involvement in the war.
- Military scouting and convoy missions during WWII were the most frequent uses for Harley-Davidson bikes. However, they were also used for other tasks, such as patrols, guard postings, and envoy jobs.
  - They appeared both on the front lines and at bases and outposts.
  - Stolen German motorcycles like BMW and Mercedes, Japanese models, Norton motorcycles, Excelsior, Indians, Triumphs, and other bikes were also used throughout the duration of the war.
  - The maneuverability and adaptability of Harley-Davidson motorcycles to a variety of terrain types made it one of the more popular bikes for the American forces in both the Pacific theater and the European and North African Campaign.
- Gasoline was a rationed item throughout the United States because of war needs.
- Aluminum became known as "unobtainium."

- The metal was being used in a variety of production of goods for the military.

- The German Wehrmacht-issued BMW R75 was one of the more powerful motorcycles at the time and had a sidecar to carry an extra soldier. The design allowed the German motorcycles to be more adaptable to different terrain types.

  - Its commanding OHV 750cc engine and design would help inspire advancements to the Harley-Davidson bikes when they were captured by the Allies.

- Police motorcycles were a way for Harley-Davidson Motor Company to grow and continue production stateside, outside of the military needs.

- In 1944, restrictions were lifted, and sales to civilians were allowed, including the sale of over 500 Knuckleheads.

  - At the same time, Harley dealers bought back surplus military bikes and sold them to customers around the country.

- Sidecar gunners were not an uncommon modification for the Harley-Davidsons used overseas.

  - Not all were equipped with a machine gun, but some were.

  - Some were set up with a mount for either a machine gun or rifle.

- o Some motorcycles were modified for transport or motorcade purposes.
- o Some simply had a setup where the person riding in the sidecar could comfortably fire their weapon depending on the position.
  - Many of these modifications were made overseas.
- There were three prototypes of the XS model that were introduced between 1941 and 1945 for the US armed forces.
  - o It was built with an opposing cylinder engine.
  - o It was designed to have dual rifle holsters and a side car.
  - o There is only one prototype left, and it currently resides in the Harley-Davidson Museum in Milwaukee.

CHAPTER 4:

POST-WORLD WAR II, THE KOREAN WAR, AND THE MOTORCYCLES OF THE '50S AND '60S

TRIVIA TIME

1. Which 1946 Harley-Davidson is considered one of the best racing motorcycles ever built?

    a. 74-cubic-inch flathead WR
    b. 45-cubic-inch flathead DL
    c. 45-cubic-inch flathead WL
    d. 45-cubic-inch flathead WR

2. Which patent were Harley-Davidson Motor Company and other Allied motorcycle businesses such as Birmingham Small Arms (BSA) able to acquire after World War II as a post-war reparation?

    a. BMW's machine gun mounts
    b. DKW's small two-stroke motor
    c. Volkswagen's OHV engine
    d. Mercedes-Benz's brake lines

3. What was the nickname of the updated one-piece rocker covers on 61 and 74-cubic-inch OHV engines with aluminum heads and hydraulic valve-lifters?

    a. "Cake-head"
    b. "Chief"
    c. "Lifter"
    d. "Panhead"

4. Hollister, California, was home to which Rally organized by the American Motorcyclist Association (AMA)?

    a. American Motorcyclist Rally
    b. Hollister Rally
    c. Gypsy Tour Motorcycle Rally
    d. Annual American Motorcycle Rally

5. In July of 1947, the small town of Hollister, California, was overwhelmed by the unexpected number of riders and motorcycles that came to their town, some of whom took things too far. After excessive imbibing of alcohol, drag races, bar fights, and vandalism, the motorcycle gathering was dubbed the Hollister Riot. What was a direct consequence of the riot?

    a. The rise of the outlaw motorcycle culture
    b. The birth of veteran culture
    c. The motorcycle saddlebag
    d. The American Motorcycle Association

6. Motorcycle clubs always had an excellent reputation in the United States in the 1950s.

a. True
b. False

7. In which year did Arthur Davidson die?

   a. 1949
   b. 1950
   c. 1955
   d. 1960

8. Which motorcycles were released during the Korean War for the American military?

   a. Model D
   b. Model UL
   c. Model WLA
   d. Model XA

9. Which motorcycle model was developed as a "kiddie" bike?

   a. Dinger
   b. Hummer
   c. Slider
   d. STU

10. Veterans returning from WWII and Korea wanted lighter motorcycles like the British twins. Which model did Harley-Davidson release in 1952 to meet this standard?

    a. F model
    b. D model
    c. K model

    d. R model

11. The hand-operated clutch appeared for the first time on which Harley-Davidson in 1952?

    a. Duo-Glide

    b. WLA

    c. Knucklehead

    d. Panhead

12. Which movie released in 1952 was inspired by the racing success of Harley-Davidson?

    a. *The Pace That Thrills*

    b. *Motorcycle Gang*

    c. *The Wild One*

    d. *One Way Ticket to Hell*

13. Harley-Davidson KR was introduced in 1953 for racing purposes.

    a. True

    b. False

14. The Sportster was first introduced in which year?

    a. 1957

    b. 1956

    c. 1955

    d. 1954

15. Which was the first (and only) scooter offered by Harley-Davidson?

    a. The Scoot

    b. The Slider

c. The Topper

d. The Bopper

16. In 1960, Harley-Davidson bought a 50% interest in Italian company Aermacchi.

    a. True

    b. False

17. What was the street bike dual sport Scrambler nicknamed?

    a. "Scat"

    b. "Rambler"

    c. "Screamer"

    d. "Mumbler"

18. Which company did Harley-Davidson purchase in 1962?

    a. Indian Motorcycle Company

    b. Tomahawk Boat Company

    c. John Deere

    d. Polaris Inc.

19. After buying the company mentioned above, which material did Harley-Davidson start using for different motorcycle parts in 1962?

    a. Polypropylene

    b. Epoxy

    c. Plexiglass

    d. Fiberglass

20. The 1965 Duo-Glide received which nickname when it was introduced with an electric starter?

    a. "Electro-Shocker"
    b. "Shock-Collar"
    c. "Electra-Glide"
    d. "Lightning Bug"

ANSWER KEY

1. D: 45-cubic-inch twins

2. B: DKW's small two-stroke motor

3. D: "Panhead"

4. C: Gypsy Tour Motorcycle Rally

5. A: The rise of the outlaw motorcycle culture

6. False

7. B: 1950

8. C: Model WLA

9. B: Hummer

10. C: Model K

11. D: Panhead

12. A: *The Pace That Thrills*

13. True

14. A: 1957

15. C: The Topper

16. True

17. A: "Scat"

18. B: Tomahawk Boat Company

19. D: Fiberglass

20. C: "Electra-glide"

FACTS, FACTOIDS, AND INTERESTING STORIES

- During campaigns in North Africa, American soldiers captured several Wehrmacht-issued motorcycles produced by BMW and Zundappas.

  o These bikes were excellent for the rough terrain of the African desert and the demands of military usage.

  o Both Harley-Davidson and Indian studied these bikes and began to develop their own versions in 1942.

    ▪ About 1,000 bikes were produced with shaft drives and flat-twin motors. They were given to the military.

      - These motorcycles cost about $35,000 each (or about a whopping $578,026 today)!

      - The information gained by studying and redesigning these motorcycles can be seen in future models.

- German patents were part of the military reparations from the war, and Harley-Davidson greatly benefited from this information.

- - Two-stroke motors from DKW were incredibly informative and useful for future production of motorcycles.
    - Model S (Hummer)
- In the year 1946, Harley-Davidson built 6,746 Knuckleheads, although they struggled to meet the demands of their customers due to shortages of materials from the war effort.
- To many, the 1947 Hollister Riot is the birthplace of the outlaw motorcycle club.
  - The most famous picture of the Hollister Riot is of a disheveled man sitting on a motorcycle drinking a bottle of beer while surrounded by discarded bottles.
    - It is theorized to have been a posed picture to make the events of the Gypsy Tour Rally and the Hollister Riot seem more shocking in order to infuriate the demure public against motorcycle enthusiasts.
- In late 1947, the Knucklehead got an overhead engine with chrome valve covers, aluminum heads, and hydraulic lifters for the OVH motor, which led to the start of the Panhead age of motorcycles for Harley-Davidson.
- Panheads and Hydra Glides were introduced during this period.

- The classic "bad boy" in films came to prominence during the 1950s, especially with the character depicted wearing a dark leather jacket and riding a motorcycle.

  o James Dean, Marlon Brando, Elvis Presley (already a big-time bad boy rock 'n' roll star in the eyes of more conservative Americans), Paul Newman, and Steve McQueen had the look that would make women swoon and men clamor to be just like them.

- The American Motorcyclist Association was originally a whites-only organization from its inception in 1924 until the mid-1950s.
- The Sportster premiered in 1957 and became a vastly popular model for the Harley-Davidson Motor Company in the coming years.
- The Duo-Glide debuted in 1957 as an advancement on the Panhead model.
- The chopper-style bike premiered in the 1950s, mainly in California. It was developed with several customizations, modifications, and changes to the standard boppers and military bikes to try to get a specific long and lean look.
- The last race of the Daytona 200 to be run on sand was won by Brad Andres.

  o 2nd–13th place was won by riders on KRs.

- The motorcycle ridden by the villain Chino (Lee Marvin's character) in the 1953 film *The Wild Ones* was either a 1949 or 1950 Flathead Bopper model.

  o All the gang members who were villains rode Indians or Harley-Davidsons.

    ▪ This did not help the reputation of the motorcycle industry or the influence of Harley-Davidson.

  o Marlon Brando's character rode a 1950 Triumph Thunderbird 6T.

- The late 1940s and early 1950s saw a shift in public perception of a Harley-Davidson (or any motorcycle for that matter) owner after the Hollister Riot.

  o The public no longer saw motorcyclists as ordinary people taking part in a variety of activities like road trips, parades, running errands, or racing. Instead, motorcyclists were viewed as drunken troublemakers.

- In 1955, Harley-Davidson released a "Wild One," an FLH Super Sport.

  o It was equipped with higher compression capacity, which bolstered the horsepower of the motorcycle by 10%.

- Servi-Car was the first Harley-Davidson model to be equipped with an electric starter in 1964.

CHAPTER 5:

THE VIETNAM WAR ERA AND THE AMF YEARS (1960S-80S)

TRIVIA TIME

1. Looking to acquire more power for their engines, Harley-Davidson Motor Company updated the design with a rocker box that looked like coal shovels for their Big Twins in 1966. What was the name of this new motor?

   a. Coalheads
   b. Shovelheads
   c. Rockerboxes
   d. Panhead 2.0

2. Which company was Harley-Davidson's biggest competition for motorcycles during the 1960s?

   a. Mitsubishi
   b. BMW
   c. Honda
   d. Ford

3. Why did Harley-Davidson need to be bought by an external company?

    a. All the Davidson family members wanted nothing to do with the company anymore
    b. The company was going bankrupt
    c. Harley-Davidson was looking to move abroad
    d. The IRS was about to charge the CFO of the company with embezzlement

4. In 1969, Harley-Davidson was publicly traded for the first time.

    a. True
    b. False

5. In which year did Harley-Davidson get bought out by American Machine and Foundry Company (AMF)?

    a. 1965
    b. 1966
    c. 1969
    d. 1970

6. AMF had previously sold which products prior to owning Harley-Davidson?

    a. Bowling balls
    b. Car parts
    c. Gun parts
    d. Electric wiring

7. What was a side effect of AMF owning Harley-Davidson?

    a. Better accessories and add-ons
    b. Better engines than ever before
    c. Nothing changed
    d. Worsening bike quality overall

8. AMF Harleys were well-loved across the board by Harley-Davidson fans.

    a. True
    b. False

9. All motorcycle clubs founded in the 1960s and 1970s were criminal "outlaw" organizations.

    a. True
    b. False

10. Which 1969 film further influenced the public's fascination with motorcycle culture, rebellious living, and the search for that elusive "something" on the open roads of the United States?

    a. *Wild Bunch*
    b. *True Grit*
    c. *The Italian Job*
    d. *Easy Rider*

11. Which style of motorcycle quickly became the quintessential bike of the "rebel" as depicted in the aforementioned movie?

    a. Bopper

b. Chopper

c. Streetfighter

d. Café Racer

12. Which new production racer was introduced by Harley-Davidson for the first time in 1970?

   a. XR-750

   b. Sportster

   c. Café Racer

   d. Mugello

13. What happened after the American Machine and Foundry Company laid off hundreds of workers from the Harley-Davidson factory?

   a. The fired workers went to work anyway

   b. The remaining workers got a pay raise

   c. Workers went on strike

   d. The fired workers sued Harley-Davidson

14. In which Pennsylvania city did Harley-Davidson open a new assembly plant in 1973?

   a. Philadelphia PA

   b. Pittsburg, PA

   c. York, PA

   d. Scranton, PA

15. What was a nickname disappointed consumers gave to the lower quality bikes of AMF Harley-Davidsons?

   a. "Hardly-Drivable"

b. "Haphazard-Drive"

c. "All Motorcycles Fail"

d. "Hellish-Disaster"

16. Motorcycles became more accessible to the American public with the rise of Japanese motorcycles of higher quality in the 1970s and into the 1980s.

a. True

b. False

17. What was the name of the 1976 American bicentennial Harley-Davidson edition?

a. The Freedom Edition

b. The Liberty Edition

c. The American Edition

d. The Yankee Edition

18. Which controversial bike model was introduced in 1977 after the bicentennial edition?

a. The Dixie Edition

b. The Rebel Edition

c. The Blue-Collar Edition

d. The Confederate Edition

19. In 1979, the Harley-Davidson Motor Company released the FXE F; what was its nickname?

a. "Fat Bob"

b. "Big Man"

c. "Little Boy"

d. "Stocky Joe"

20. With regard to Harley-Davidson Motor Company, what did AMF do in 1981?

    a. Bought Indian Motorcycle Company and combined the two for just under $90 million
    b. Shut down all of its international offices to save $450 million
    c. Sold the company to thirteen investors, including Vaughn Beals, for about $75 million
    d. Shut down the company for a $100 million refurbishment project

ANSWER KEY

1. B: Shovelheads

2. C: Honda

3. B: The company was going bankrupt

4. True

5. C: 1969

6. A: Bowling balls

7. D: Worsening bike quality

8. False

9. False

10. D: *Easy Rider*

11. B: Chopper

12. A: XR-750

13. C: Workers went on strike

14. C: York, PA

15. A: "Hardly-Drivable"

16. True

17. B: The Liberty Edition

18. D: The Confederate Edition

19. A: "Fat Bob"

20. C: Sold the company to thirteen investors, including Vaughn Beals, for about $75 million

FACTS, FACTOIDS, AND INTERESTING STORIES

- Military Police were the most common riders of Harley-Davidsons during the Vietnam War and the Cold War era, although there were several instances of Harley-Davidsons and other motorcycles being used in envoy and reconnaissance missions.
- The FXEF "Fat Bob" model was introduced in 1979 and had dual gas tanks and bobbed fenders.
  - o The "Fat Bob" model contributed in part to the "Fat Boy" model.
- Vietnam veterans were the leading number of individuals to found and/or join motorcycle clubs upon returning home from the war after military service. They began riding their motorcycles across the country.
  - o A portion of those motorcycle clubs had been founded after the Second World War by the veterans returning home from North Africa, Europe, and Southeast Asia.
  - o After taking part in the Vietnam War, many veterans felt lost and disenfranchised from conflicting anti-war/warmongering ideologies.
  - o Of those clubs they joined, a handful were "outlaw" clubs.

- *Easy Rider* (1969) featured one of the most famous motorcycles in the world, and it became the prototypical motorcycle of the counterculture/rebel.
- In 1973, AMF noted they would be moving some production plants from Milwaukee, Wisconsin, to York, Pennsylvania.
  - o It turned out that only engines would continue to be produced in Milwaukee while all the other parts would be made in York.
  - o The company infamously promised the workers' unions they were not going to fire any laborers during their moving process and then promptly let many workers go.
    - ▪ The workers felt betrayed by the company's lies in failing to uphold their word with their employees.
      - Those that were awaiting either their pink slips or a potential pay cut stated their prediction that the "Milwaukee Hog" would become "York Pork."
- HAWG, or the Harley Action Workers Group, was formed in the early 1970s after the changeover of factory locations.
  - o Members started a campaign of refusing to work overtime to carry out a passive resistance to the AMF.

- Some Harley-Davidson employees took a more aggressive approach to the AMF's efforts and carried out a tradition of many past jilted factory workers: sabotaging production.
- In 1974, AMF promised to invest $5.5 million in equipment in the Milwaukee plant as a show of faith and to help with production problems.
  - AMF failed to negotiate with the unions, leading to further frustrations and a workers' strike.
    - The strike ended in September of 1974 once the AMF finally agreed to the workers' demands to make the promised 1975 line of motorcycles and meet their quota.
- Despite all the issues with AMF bikes, collectors love to acquire AMF-era Harley-Davidsons.
  - The 1977 Café Racer XLCR is considered a highly sought-after model.
    - Willie G. Davidson, a direct grandson of one of the Davidson brothers, designed the XLCR.
    - Only 3,100 were sold.
    - It was discontinued in 1978.
- FXS Lowrider was introduced in the year 1977.

CHAPTER 6:

AFTER THE AMF AND THE 1990S

TRIVIA TIME

1. What was one of the fundamentals that the new company executives of Harley-Davidson planned to carry out to help with the corporate turnaround following the purchase from AMF in 1981?

    a. Implement quality control
    b. Buy new parts for production
    c. Sell to another parent company
    d. Invest in stock

2. Which model was introduced in 1982?

    a. XLCR Café Racer
    b. FXE "Fat Bob"
    c. FXR Super Glide II
    d. FXS Low Rider

3. What was the motto associated with the Harley-Davidson manufacturing inventory system in 1982?

    a. "Here We Go"
    b. "Nick-of-Time"

c. "Fast and Furious"

d. "Just-in-Time"

4. Which group was formed in 1983?

   a. Motorcyclists Organization Group (MOG)

   b. Small Motorcycles Owners Group (SMOG)

   c. Dealers and Owners Group (DOG)

   d. Harley Owners Group (HOG)

5. What did the above group petition the International Trade Commission (ITC) to impose in 1983?

   a. Tariffs on other American motorcycles over 500cc

   b. Tariffs on Japanese motorcycles over 700cc

   c. Tariffs on British motorcycles over 700cc

   d. Tariffs on Italian motorcycles over 750cc

6. Which engine appeared in five Harley-Davidson models in 1984?

   a. 1340cc V2 Evolution engine

   b. 450cc Flathead V-twin engine

   c. 750cc Class C flathead engine

   d. "F-Head" single-cylinder engine

7. What was the name of the Harley-Davidsons that included a concealed rear suspension and a rigid frame designed to appear like the older models?

   a. Old Fashioned

   b. Hard-Frame

   c. Softail

   d. Rough Rider

8. The aforementioned model with the concealed rear suspension was an economic failure for Harley-Davidson.

    a. True
    b. False

9. Which company did the Harley-Davidson Motor Company acquire in 1986 to diversify its production of products?

    a. Volkswagen
    b. Indian Motorcycle Company
    c. Holiday Rambler Motorhome Company
    d. Jayco, Inc.

10. During its Initial Public Offering (IPO), Harley-Davidson debuted on the New York Stock Exchange (NYSE) under which ticker symbol?

    a. SPF (Scrambler Proprietors Firm)
    b. MCC (Motorcycle Club Company)
    c. HDMC (Harley-Davidson Motorcycle Company)
    d. HOG (Harley Owners Group)

11. The Harley-Davidson Motor Company petitioned the International Trade Commission to alleviate the previously negotiated levy on imported motorcycles a year before its lapse in 1987 to allow for a more level playing field.

    a. True
    b. False

12. Japanese motorcycle companies began producing V-twin cruisers in 1987.

    a. True

    b. False

13. Which motorcycle was introduced in 1990?

    a. FXEF "Fat Boy"

    b. XLCR "Café Racer"

    c. FLSTF "Fat Boy"

    d. FLT

14. What was the name of the new line introduced in 1991?

    a. Springer

    b. Dyna

    c. Fat Man

    d. Legacy

15. By 1992, save for a few racing bikes, Harley-Davidson became the first company to equip all their bikes with which of the following?

    a. V2 twin engines

    b. Foot brakes

    c. GPS systems

    d. Drive belts

16. In 1993, which motorcycle company did Harley-Davidson Motor Company purchase minority shares in?

    a. Triumph Motorcycle Company

b. Honda Motorcycle Company

c. Buell Motorcycle Company

d. Indian Motorcycle Company

17. Which water-cooled Harley-Davidson motorcycle entered the AMA Superbike Championship in Poland in 1994?

    a. DOHC VR1000

    b. FLSTF "Fat Boy"

    c. FXDB Dyna Glide

    d. FX1200 Super Glide

18. Which new feature was equipped for the first time on the new models of Harley-Davidson motorcycles in 1995?

    a. A U-shaped seat

    b. Fuel injection

    c. Windshields

    d. "Sissy bars"

19. Where did Harley-Davidson open a new 217,000square-foot design center in 1997?

    a. Indianapolis, Indiana

    b. St. Petersburg, Florida

    c. Chicago, Illinois

    d. Milwaukee, Wisconsin

20. In 1998, where did Harley-Davidson open its first foreign factory?

    a. Manaus, Brazil

    b. Berlin, Germany

c. Lisbon, Portugal
d. Bangkok, Thailand

ANSWER KEY

1. A: Implement quality control

2. C: FXR Super Glide II

3. D: "Just-in-Time"

4. D: Harley Owners Group (HOG)

5. B: Tariffs on Japanese motorcycles over 700cc

6. A: 1340cc V2 Evolution engine

7. C: Softail

8. False

9. C: Holiday Rambler Motorhome Company

10. D: HOG (Harley Owners Group)

11. True

12. True

13. C: FLSTF "Fat Boy"

14. B: Dyna

15. D: Drive belts

16. C: Buell Motorcycle Company

17. A: DOHC VR1000

18. B: Fuel injection

19. D: Milwaukee, Wisconsin

20. A: Manaus, Brazil

FACTS, FACTOIDS, AND INTERESTING STORIES

- The mismanagement of the AMF-owned Harley-Davidson Motor Company resulted in some of the worst years for the company, losing nearly all of its loyal customers and leaving profits in freefall.
- In 1983, Harley introduced the Sportster model with a different style.
  - It became known as a Sportster XLX-61.
    - It came with low bars, a peanut tank, and a solo seat.
    - With little chrome and only available in black, this model became incredibly popular due to its power and low price of $3,995 (about $10,700 today).
- The Softail model received a new frame in 1984.
- In 1984, the Evolution engine was introduced.
- The "Just-in-Time" inventory system adopted by Harley-Davidson Motor Company in 1982 had achieved both a lower cost and an increase in the quality of the manufactured goods following the corporation's independence from AMF management.
- Because of the public's love of the old-school styling of the Springer, 1988 saw the return of the

traditional front end on the new FXSTS Springer Softails.

- ○ The Springer fork reappeared in 1988.
- The Big Twins motorcycles got a profiled belt in place of the starter pedal in 1986.
- With the 1983 petition to the International Trade Commission, Harley-Davidson wanted the ITC to impose a tariff on Japanese motorcycles over 700cc, which had been sleeved down in the U.S. from its traditional 750cc (as it was sold elsewhere around the globe).
- The FLSTF Fat Boy was introduced in 1990.
- In 1991, the first of the Dyna line was the FXDB Dyna Glide Sturgis.
- Drive belts, which became the standard for most Harley-Davidson motorcycles except for a handful of the racing models, provided a much smoother ride compared to models with chains.

    ○ The drive belts lasted longer and did not necessitate frequent adjustments or oil lubrication as the chains required.

- Harley-Davidson premiered the water-cooled DOHC VR1000 at the 1994 AMA Superbike Championship in Poland.

    ○ The riders who took part in the race were Scott Russell, Miguel Duhamel, Pascal Picotte, and Chris Carr.

- AMA rules required Harley to 'construct and sell 2,000 models for road use.
  - Procedures and regulations were more lenient in Poland, allowing for scarcely adapted motorcycles to be authorized and certified to compete.
  - None of the VR1000 ever won in the AMA race.
- The Electra Glide Ultra Classic implemented the electronic injection from the Magneti Marelli in 1995.
- In 1995, Harley-Davidson first introduced fuel injection, which would become incredibly popular for their bikes.
- By 1996, the sale of parts and accessories became equally important to Harley-Davidson Motor Company as selling motorcycles, so improvements and growth were vital for the business's success.
  - They opened a 250,000-square-foot facility in Franklin, Wisconsin.
- In 1997, FL engine production moved to a new plant in Menomonee Falls, Wisconsin, around the same time that a new design center opened in Milwaukee.
  - They also built a 330,000-square-foot facility in Kansas City, Missouri, to take over all production of the Sportsters.
- Harley-Davidson acquired the remaining shares of Buell in 1998.

CHAPTER 7:

THE END OF THE '90S, INTO THE AUGHTS

TRIVIA TIME

1. In 1999, which new engines did the Dyna and Touring lines receive?

   a. Side-valve engines
   b. V-twin engines
   c. Twin Cam88 engine
   d. 1340cc V2 Evolution engine

2. Which sound did Harley-Davidson try to trademark through the U.S. Patent Office?

   a. Rum-Rum-Rum-Rum
   b. Potato-Potato
   c. Bbbrrr-Bbbrrr-Bbbrrr
   d. Plumb-Plumb-Plumb

3. Harley-Davidson had spent thousands of dollars throughout the mid-90s on legal fees for the previously mentioned trademark sound.

   a. True
   b. False

4. The patent application was eventually dropped in 2000 despite this engine's reverberation being a greatly loved and revered sound favored by Harley-Davidson enthusiasts.

   a. True
   b. False

5. Which model was introduced in 2001?

   a. FXDB Dyna Glide
   b. Rambler 2001
   c. WLDR
   d. VRSC V-Rod

6. Which famous car company provided input for the fuel-injected motor of the model introduced in 2001?

   a. Lamborghini
   b. Porsche
   c. BMW
   d. Jaguar

7. How many people are estimated to have traveled to Milwaukee, Wisconsin, to attend Harley-Davidson Motor Company's 100th Anniversary in 2003?

   a. 250,000
   b. 350,000
   c. 420,000
   d. 500,000

8. In 2006, which huge pronouncement did Harley-Davidson Motor Company make about the corporation's future?

a. Harley-Davidson Motor Company was selling half of its investments back to AMF.
b. Harley-Davidson Motor Company was publicshing a new magazine.
c. Harley-Davidson planned to open a new museum in Milwaukee.
d. Harley-Davidson Motor Company declared bankruptcy and the intent to shut down factories.

9. After the '06 Dyna model first debuted this feature, what became a standard transmission for all Dyna models across the board in 2007?

   a. Three-speed transmission
   b. Four-speed transmission
   c. Five-speed transmission
   d. Six-speed transmission

10. After the updates were made to the 2007 Twin motors, what were they stoked out to be?

   a. 80 cubic inches
   b. 92 cubic inches
   c. 96 cubic inches
   d. 100 cubic inches

11. What was the nickname given to these new motors?

   a. Twin Cam 92
   b. Twin Cam 96
   c. Twin Cam 80

d. Twin Cam 100

12. On its 105th Anniversary in 2008, Harley-Davidson opened its impressive museum.

    a. True
    b. False

13. In 2008, Harley-Davidson purchased the MV Agusto for $109 million to try to achieve what?

    a. Take advantage of the lack of sales abroad
    b. Kill the company
    c. Sell more off-road bikes
    d. Benefit from the MV European distribution networks

14. Which model of motorcycle was introduced in 2008?

    a. FLT
    b. FLSTF "Fat Boy"
    c. XR1200
    d. Duo-Glide

15. The first motorcycle to be debuted by Harley-Davidson in Japan was the XR750 flat track machine.

    a. True
    b. False

16. In 2009, who was the first person since 1981 to become CEO of Harley-Davidson without any prior connection to the company?

    a. Joanne B. Schmann
    b. Keith Wandell

c. Danny Eslick
d. Scott Russell

17. What caused Harley-Davidson to stop production of the Buell line?

    a. Harley-Davidson stock surged, and they didn't need Buell
    b. Buell merged with Triumph
    c. Harley-Davidson sold Buell to Honda
    d. The Recession

18. What did Harley-Davidson do to focus on its core business in 2009?

    a. Sold all its holdings in Holiday Rambler
    b. Invested in aluminum and other metals
    c. Put MV Agusto up for sale
    d. Bought more land to build more factories

19. Why did Harley have to focus its business in 2009?

    a. The company declared an 84% drop in profit
    b. Avoid bankruptcy
    c. Investment opportunities in foreign companies
    d. 72% European market growth

20. In the same year, Harley-Davidson planned to enter the Indian market, as it was becoming increasingly profitable.

    a. True
    b. False

ANSWER KEY

1. C: Twin Cam88 Engines

2. B: Potato-Potato

3. True

4. True

5. D: VRSC V-Rod

6. B: Porsche

7. A: 250,000

8. C: Harley-Davidson announced its intention to open a brand-new museum in Milwaukee, Wisconsin, in the upcoming years.

9. D: Six-speed transmission

10. C: 96 cubic inches

11. B: Twin Cam 96

12. True

13. D: Attempt to benefit from the MV European distribution networks

14. C: XR1200

15. False

16. B: Keith Wandell

17. D: The Recession

18. C: Put MV Agusto up for sale

19. A: The company declared an 84% drop in profit

20. True

FACTS, FACTOIDS, AND INTERESTING STORIES

- At the start of the new millennium, Harley-Davidson spent tens of thousands of dollars in legal fees trying to patent the potato-potato sound of the Harley motor but eventually dropped the application after several years of difficulty.

  o Joanne Bischmann, the Vice President of Marketing, said, "I've personally spoken with Harley-Davidson owners from around the world, and they've told me repeatedly there is nothing like the sound of a Harley-Davidson motorcycle. If our customers know the sound cannot be imitated, that's good enough for me and for Harley-Davidson."

- Porsche gave input for the motor of the new VRSC V-Rod, which debuted in 2001.

  o This included the overhead camshaft and liquid cooling.

- The '06 model year Dyna motorcycles came with a six-speed transmission, and they quickly became the standard for the models with the Twin Cam 96 after 2006.

- In 2004, all four founding members of Harley-Davidson Motor Company — William Davidson, Walter Davidson, William Harley, and Arthur

Davidson—were inducted into the Labor Hall of Fame for their contributions to workers and for their efforts for the company.

- Harley introduced the XR1200 in 2008, which was inspired by the XR750 flat track machine.
  - o It was used to win many championships for Harley-Davidson.
  - o The XR1200 became the first Harley-Davidson to be promoted and constructed exclusively for the European market.
- Brazil, Thailand, and India all produced Harley-Davidsons.
- In 2006, the Harley-Davidson ticker logo was changed on the New York Stock Exchange from HDI to HOG.
- The 2008 Recession contributed heavily to many of the changes for Harley-Davidson in the late aughts that impacted the company for years to come.
- The Indian market became incredibly important to the recovery from the 2008 Recession for the Harley-Davidson Motor Company.
  - o It was exceedingly difficult for the company to sink its teeth into the Indian market due to the high taxes and tariffs on foreign goods.

CHAPTER 8:

2010S TO THE PRESENT

TRIVIA TIME

1. Harley-Davidson Motor Company restructured in 2010.

    a. True
    b. False

2. Harley-Davidson Motor Company demanded the labor unions in Wisconsin acquiesce to compromises on three seven-year-long contracts permitting $50 million dollars in savings in labor costs.

    a. True
    b. False

3. How many factory jobs were lost in the factories and assembly plants in Milwaukee and Tomahawk because of the restructuring?

    a. 623 jobs
    b. 502 jobs
    c. 481 jobs
    d. 375 jobs

4. The assembly plant for Harley-Davidson in Kansas City, Missouri, is one of the most active motorcycle factories in the country today.

   a. True
   b. False

5. To avoid having to pay import tariffs in India, where did Harley open an assembly plant?

   a. Delhi
   b. Kolkata
   c. Bawal
   d. Mumbai

6. Who broke the 1999 long-distance motorcycle jump record in 2011?

   a. Roger Craig Knievel
   b. Bubba Blackwell
   c. Erik Buell
   d. Seth Enslow

7. What was that record?

   a. 194.5 feet
   b. 149.2 feet
   c. 183.7 feet
   d. 134.6 feet

8. Which model was set for customization in 2011, permitting buyers to get factory-constructed specialty motorcycles?

   a. H-D1

b. Softail Slim
c. Fat Bob
d. Flathead

9. Between 2000 and 2013, how many motorcycle riders were officially trained to ride through the New Rider's Course of the River's Edge Harley-Davidson Academy of Motorcycling?

    a. 200,000 riders
    b. 300,000 riders
    c. 400,000 riders
    d. 500,000 riders

10. In 2014, what was the name of the project that was developed to use focus groups, customer workshops, and other external contributions to help design new projects?

    a. Harley Customs
    b. Lincoln
    c. Rushmore
    d. HD Consumer Projection

11. Which Marvel character rode a 2014 model Harley-Davidson Street 750 in two different *Avengers* films?

    a. Carol Danvers, Captain Marvel
    b. James Buchanan "Bucky" Barnes, the Winter Soldier
    c. Peter Quill, Star Lord
    d. Steve Rogers, Captain America

12. Which other Marvel character rode a prototype of an electric Harley-Davidson, called Project LiveWire, in the 2015 film *Avengers: Age of Ultron*?

    a. Wanda Maximoff, Scarlet Witch
    b. Clint Barton, Hawkeye
    c. Natasha Romanoff, Black Widow
    d. Sam Wilson, Falcon

13. Which toy company introduced a model of the Harley-Davidson Fat Boy?

    a. Little Tikes
    b. Hasbro
    c. LEGO
    d. Playmobile

14. Project LiveWire was a rounding success, with profits exceeding all expectations.

    a. True
    b. False

15. In 2017, Harley-Davidson Motor Company distributed over 241,000 bikes to dealerships around the United States. How did this number of motorcycles fair in comparison to other years of shipments?

    a. Lowest in the company's history
    b. On average
    c. Lowest in six years
    d. Highest in ten years

16. Harley-Davidson was forced to close its factory in which city in 2018?

    a. Milwaukee, Wisconsin
    b. York, Pennsylvania
    c. Detroit, Michigan
    d. Kansas City, Missouri

17. Which material was affected by the $30 million U.S. import tariff tax in 2018?

    a. Steel
    b. Leather
    c. Chrome
    d. Plastics

18. The millennial and Z generations are the top national consumers of Harley-Davidsons because the bikes are cheap, averaging $10,000, including accessories and customizations.

    a. True
    b. False

19. Due to the COVID-19 pandemic, Harley-Davidson saw an increase in sales and profit.

    a. True
    b. False

20. How did Harley-Davidson launch their 2021 line to celebrate their 118th birthday in February 2021?

    a. Block party at the original site of the factory in Milwaukee, Wisconsin

b. Free giveaways of accessory products at all national distributors
c. Debuted the entire 2022 line
d. Hosted an online virtual event

ANSWER KEY

1. True

2. True

3. D: 375 jobs

4. False

5. C: Bawal

6. D: Seth Enslow

7. C: 183.7 feet

8. A: H-D1

9. B': 300,000 Riders

10. C: Rushmore

11. D: Steve Rogers, Captain America

12. C: Natasha Romanoff, Black Widow

13. C: LEGO

14. False

15. C: Lowest in six years

16. D: Kansas City Missouri

17. A: Steel

18. False

19. False

20. D: Hosted an online virtual event

FACTS, FACTOIDS, AND INTERESTING STORIES

- Harley-Davidson had a rough decade because of the Recession and, most recently, due to COVID-19, which has caused many losses for the company.

  o Fewer motorcycles have been sold.

- Recalls for motorcycles have become incredibly common in the past few years, and Harley-Davidson suffered a lot of losses.

  o In 2018, under 240,000 Harley-Davidson motorcycles were recalled because of a clutch deficiency, which cost $35,000,000.

  o Harley stopped production on the Street model in 2019 when it recalled over 44,0000 bikes for a defective brake.

- The Harley-Davidson Bawal factory officially closed its doors in 2020, having suffered the effects of COVID-19 and trouble breaking out into the market.

  o Harley-Davidson followed the move of General Motors, which had departed from the Indian market in 2017.

  o Ford left India in 2019.

- o Toyota stated their intention to halt their expansion plans in India, citing the taxes they were facing.

  - India is known for its high taxes and tariffs, especially on foreign products and companies.

- Harley-Davidson is facing the difficulty of having its clientele grow older. The company also struggled in the Recession, post-Recession, and COVID years.

- LiveWire, despite being an excellent premiere with fans of electric motorcycles, did poorly, and Harley-Davidson was unable to market it to customers.

  - o It was one of the worst releases for Harley-Davidson.
  - o It had a high price tag and did not have the revolutionary results the company had hoped for.

- Harley-Davidson Motor Company has gone through many years of transition and continues to adapt to the changing times.

- Overseas, Harley-Davidsons are not as popular as European or Asian models, and sales continue to struggle abroad.

- Harley-Davidson production has cut down significantly in recent years, and fewer new bikes are being made in the United States (or anywhere for that matter).

- COVID-19 has severely impacted Harley-Davidson production and dealerships.

- Harley-Davidson had always been a symbol of rebellion, especially in the conservative 1950s, but in recent years, Harley-Davidsons no longer have that image for those seeking to "fight the man."
- Harley-Davidson has received a lot of heat from some more "patriotic" Americans for producing their motorcycles overseas, although most Harley owners and riders have not stated one way or another whether they were upset.
- Harley-Davidsons are one of the most popular bikes in the world.

  - Statistically, however, these bikes are most frequently bought by the Baby Boomer Generation and Generation X.
  - Younger generations frequently own foreign bikes such as Triumph, Suzuki, BMW, Indian, and Honda.

CHAPTER 9:

HARLEY-DAVIDSON IN STUNTS, FILMS, TELEVISION, AND THE MEDIA

TRIVIA TIME

1. Which Harley-Davidson model appears in the 1924 Buster Keaton film *Sherlock Jr.*, featuring one of the most famous stunts and motorcycle scenes in film history?

    a. Model A
    b. Flathead
    c. Panhead
    d. Model J

2. What was a popular manner of publicizing Harley-Davidsons in the 1930s?

    a. Stickers
    b. Advertisements
    c. Books
    d. Cartoons

3. The 1964 film *Roustabout* featured Elvis Presley riding a 1958 Panhead FHL Duo Glide.

   a. True
   b. False

4. Which James Bond film famously featured villains pursuing the super spy on their Aermacchi Harley-Davidson 350 SS motorcycles?

   a. *Dr. No*
   b. *On Her Majesty's Secret Service*
   c. *Live and Let Die*
   d. *Goldfinger*

5. Sylvester Stallone rode a 1978 FLH Electra Glide in which film?

   a. *Rocky III*
   b. *First Blood*
   c. *Rocky IV*
   d. *Stop! Or My Mom Will Shoot!*

6. Which Harley-Davidson successfully jumped over nineteen cars in Ontario, California, and was featured in the 1971 film *Evel Knievel*?

   a. Model D
   b. XR-750 Iron Head
   c. FXD Street Bob
   d. Panhead

7. *Every Which Way but Loose* featured, which fictional gang riding Harley-Davidsons?

a. "The Rabid Dogs"
b. "The One-Eyed Snakes"
c. "The Lizards of the West"
d. "The Black Widows"

8. Harley-Davidsons were exclusively used in all of Evel Knievel's motorcycle stunts.

   a. True
   b. False

9. Which model of Harley-Davidson was the motorcycle of choice for Robocop in the 1990 flick *Robocop 2*?

   a. Fat Boy
   b. FXSTC Softail Custom
   c. FXR Super Glide
   d. FLH Electra Glide

10. Arnold Schwarzenegger reprised his role of the T-800 Terminator in 1991's *Terminator 2: Judgement Day* in his motorcycle jacket, leather pants, and biker boots. Which 1990 model Harley-Davidson made an appearance in the iconic chase scene involving a Harley, a Honda motorbike, and a Freightliner truck?

    a. Panhead Chopper
    b. Sportster
    c. Fat Boy
    d. Hydra-Glide

11. The 1991 film *Harley-Davidson and the Marlboro Man* features which motorcycle?

a. 1989 FXR Super Glide II
b. 1989 Knucklehead
c. 1989 Hydra Glide
d. 1989 FXLR

12. Which 1994 Quentin Tarantino film featured a 1986 FXR Super Glide named Grace, a samurai sword, and a gold pocket watch in one of the movie's more infamous vignettes?

a. *Reservoir Dogs*
b. *Kill Bill vol. 2*
c. *Jackie Brown*
d. *Pulp Fiction*

13. Which X-Men character is often depicted riding a motorcycle in the comic books?

a. Cyclops
b. Wolverine
c. Mystique
d. Sabretooth

14. The 2007 *Ghost Rider* film starring Nicholas Cage featured which model of a custom Harley-Davidson?

a. Street Bob
b. Street Glide
c. Panhead Chopper
d. Softail

15. Which 2008 sequel to a popular movie franchise featured the character Mutt Williams riding a 1942 WLA Harley-Davidson Softail Springer Classic?

a. *Indiana Jones and the Kingdom of the Crystal Skull*
b. *The Mummy: Tomb of the Dragon Emperor*
c. *Rambo*
d. *Hellboy II: The Golden Army*

16. Jackson "Jax" Teller was the main character in the show *Sons of Anarchy* about a fictional outlaw motorcycle club in California. Which Harley-Davidson did the character ride throughout most of the show?

    a. 2003 Dyna Super Glide Sport
    b. 2005 Panhead
    c. 2011 FXD Street Bob
    d. Custom Chopper

17. What is the name of the *Sons of Anarchy* spinoff show that debuted in 2018, which featured many different Harley-Davidson motorcycle models, including the FLSTN Softail Deluxe, Dyna Super Glide Sport, Heritage Softail, Dyna Street Bob, Road King, and Panhead?

    a. *The Sons Ride Again*
    b. *Mayans, MC*
    c. *The Banditos*
    d. *Devil's Tribe, MC*

18. What is the nickname associated with the Shovelhead Chopper featured in the 2008 film *Hell Ride*?

    a. "The Burnout"
    b. "The Red Man"

c. "The Fella"

d. "The Gent"

19. Which Harley-Davidson motorcycle did Jax Teller restore and then ride in the final scene of *Sons of Anarchy*?

    a. 1985 FXR Chopper

    b. 2011 FXD Street Bob

    c. 1946 Custom EL Knucklehead

    d. 1968 Custom Chopper

20. The 2016 show *Harley and Davidsons* is a documentary series based on the company. It used film and shots from archive footage to tell the history of the business and its founders.

    a. True

    b. False

ANSWER KEY

1. D: Model J

2. B: Advertisements

3. False

4. C: *Live and Let Die*

5. A: *Rocky III*

6. B: XR-750 Iron Head

7. C: "The Black Widows"

8. False

9. B: FXSTC Softail Custom

10. C: Fat Boy

11. D: 1989 FXLR

12. D: *Pulp Fiction*

13. B: Wolverine

14. C: Panhead Chopper

15. A: *Indiana Jones and the Kingdom of the Crystal Skull*

16. A: 2003 Dyna Super Glide Sport

17. B: *Mayans, MC*

18. D: "The Gent"

19. C: 1946 Custom EL Knucklehead

20. False

FACTS, FACTOIDS, AND INTERESTING STORIES

- The Buster Keaton film *Sherlock Jr.* featured a stunt that became one of the most famous scenes involving a Harley-Davidson and one of the most impressive stunts ever performed on film.

  o In the scene, Buster Keaton rides on the front of a motorcycle. The driver falls off when they pass through a mud puddle, and he continues to ride the vehicle without the driver.

    ▪ Keaton inadvertently rides across a collapsing bridge, goes through some farms, drives over two trucks knocks down a stag party, nearly avoids hitting many people and items, weaves between many cars and streetcars, avoids a train, and traverses a series of different terrain, including some woods, a stream, and city streets.

    ▪ Buster Keaton suffered several injuries because of his stunts in the film.

- The 1978 Clint Eastwood film *Every Which Way but Loose* and its 1980 sequel *Every Which Way You Can* featured bare-knuckle boxing, an orangutan, and a hilariously incompetent revenge-seeking motorcycle gang called the "Black Widows," who spent most of the film trying to beat up the hero.

- The gang rode multiple Harley-Davidsons, including a couple of Sportsters, an Electra Glide, and a Panhead.
  - There were also a few choppers and a couple of sidecars featured.
- In George A. Romero's 1978 *Dawn of the Dead*, a sequel to his 1968 low-budget horror film *Night of the Living Dead*, a gang of malicious bikers under the command of biker Blade, played by Romero's good friend and actor/makeup legend Tom Savini, raid the mall where the protagonists are hiding out, bringing with them zombies and destruction.
  - They ride in on many different Harley-Davidsons, including a 1973 Aermacchi Harley-Davidson RCX 125, a Harley-Davidson Panhead Chopper, a Shovelhead, a 1977 Harley-Davidson FX Super Glide, Panheads, a Harley Servi-Car, a 1977 Harley-Davidson 1200 Super Glide, Choppers, and a 1969 Harley-Davidson FL Electra Glide.
- In the 1992 David Lynch film *Twin Peaks: Fire Walk with Me*, one of the protagonists drives a 1975 Harley-Davidson Electra Glide.
- In the rebooted BBC's *Dr. Who* series, a FLSTC Heritage Softail Classic appeared in a few episodes.
- George A. Romero, best known for founding the zombie horror genre with his Night of the Living

Dead film series, directed the 1981 film about motorcycle jousting crews, *Knightriders*.

- o Although it is one of the most famous motorcycle movies ever made, it did not feature any Harleys, but instead Yamahas and Hondas.
  - ▪ It also featured a cameo by Stephen King.
- Harley-Davidson also made an appearance in the 2018 film *Pacific Rim: Uprising* and the 2019 Marvel film *Captain Marvel*.
  - o Both featured a Harley-Davidson XL1000 Sportster.
- Action star and bodybuilding legend Arnold Schwarzenegger has collected multiple models of motorcycles, including a Fat Boy FLSTF, among his most well-recognized and best-remembered bikes.
- The 1973 film *Electra Glide in Blue* featured actor Robert Blake as the character John Wintergreen; a disillusioned cop put on a demanding highway to deal with the rough individuals and criminal entities as a traffic cop after a difficult stint as a homicide policeman.
  - o He rode a Harley-Davidson Shovelhead FL Electra Glide.
- Stephen King, who is known for his cameos in the film and television adaptations of his books such as *IT Chapter 2*, *The Stand*, and *Creepshow*, rode a red Harley-Davidson Road Glide in his guest appearance on the show *Sons of Anarchy*, although

he had always stated his adoration for his 1986 Heritage Soft Tail.

- Harley-Davidson played an important yet understated role in the show *Sons of Anarchy*, which featured many different classic and new Harley-Davidsons, including Road Kings, Dyna Super Glide Sports, Dyna Wideglides, Heritage Softails, Dyna Street Bobs, a Panhead, Custom Choppers, Lowrider Softail, Knuckleheads, Fat Bobs, Softails, Screamin' Eagle Road King, and an Electra Tri-Glide.
- In the *Machete* series, starring Danny Trejo, he is featured atop a Softail outfitted with a minigun.

  o Who does not want one of those when they hit some terrible traffic and have to deal with road rage?

CHAPTER 10:

MOTORCYCLE CLUBS, CRIMINAL MOTORCYCLE GANGS, AND THE HARLEY-DAVIDSON

TRIVIA TIME

1. What is the name of the first Motorcycle Club founded in 1903?
   a. Hell's Angels, MC
   b. Nomads, MC
   c. Outlaws, MC
   d. Yonkers, MC

2. Which event, which heavily featured Harley-Davidson motorcycles, is considered to be the catalyst to the birth of the 1%-er American outlaw motorcycle club culture?
   a. World War I
   b. The Death of Walter Davidson
   c. The Hollister Riot
   d. The Korean War

3. What does M.C. stand for?

   a. Motorized Car
   b. Motorbike Carriers
   c. Motorcycle Club
   d. Motor Captain

4. What percentage of motorcycle gangs are said to be criminal?

   a. 1%
   b. 5%
   c. 30%
   d. 100%

5. Veterans of World War II looked to recapture the camaraderie of military service, which helped contribute to the growth of motorcycle gangs and motorcycle clubs across the country. Men returning from North Africa, Europe, and the Pacific sought to recapture the brotherhood of the military and the rush of battle, embracing a nomadic life of uncertainty on the open road.

   a. True
   b. False

6. All motorcycle clubs are criminal.

   a. True
   b. False

7. There were only two motorcycle clubs at the beginning of the post-World War II era.

a. True
b. False

8. Which American Motorcyclist Association event held at Hollister, California, in 1947 is credited with the birth of the motorcycle gang?

   a. Hollister Rally
   b. California Motorist Rally
   c. American Motorcyclist Association Rally
   d. Gypsy Tour Motorcycle Rally

9. Which term associated with criminal motorcycle gangs distinguishes them from the rest of the motorcycle clubs that exist around the world?

   a. Villains
   b. Thieves
   c. Outlaws
   d. Fugitives

10. Motorcycle clubs are exclusively found in the United States.

    a. True
    b. False

11. What was a contributing factor, aside from being American-made and a vehicle that American World War II veterans were familiar with, that made the Harley-Davidson a vital motivation purchase by motorcycle clubs?

    a. No foreign motorcycles were being imported.

b. Harley-Davidson advertised exclusively to military veterans and motorcycle clubs.

c. Harley-Davidson Motor Company gave discounts to groups.

d. Harley-Davidsons were cheaper than foreign imported motorcycles.

12. Which motorcycle gang took part in a fight that broke out at the 1969 Altamont concert during the performance of the Rolling Stones and led to the death of one person?

    a. Banditos
    b. Galloping Goose
    c. Hell's Angels
    d. Pagans

13. What are the vests worn by many motorcycle clubs and gangs called?

    a. Vests
    b. Kuttes (Cuts)
    c. Shirts
    d. Leathers

14. Motorcycle clubs, especially criminal ones, tend to be divided by sex and race, although there are some exceptions.

    a. True
    b. False

15. Which one of these outlaw motorcycle clubs is not real but featured in the American animated television show *Bob's Burgers*?

    a. Outlaws
    b. Warlocks
    c. One-Eyed Snakes
    d. Sons of Silence

16. Who wrote the 1967 book *Hell's Angels: The Strange and Terrible Saga of the Outlaw Motorcycle Gangs* that featured an incredibly comprehensive and harsh examination of the outlaw motorcycle club?

    a. S.E. Hinton
    b. John Steinbeck
    c. Jack Kerouac
    d. Hunter S. Thompson

17. How long did the aforementioned author spend with the Hell's Angels to be able to acquire a better understanding of the outlaw motorcycle club?

    a. One week
    b. One month
    c. One summer
    d. One year

18. Geographic locations such as regions or states can be used as distinctive markers for certain outlaw motorcycle clubs and gangs. When one crosses that line or challenges another's "territory," this can lead to violence amongst the different associations.

a. True
b. False

19. What is the name of the Harley-Davidson–sanctioned coalition that is designed to help build a community of Harley-Davidson motorcycle owners?

   a. Harley-Davidson Confederation (HDC)
   b. Harley Motorcyclists Association (HMA)
   c. Harley Owners Group (HOG)
   d. Harley-Davidson Organization (HDO)

20. How many official chapters of this Harley-Davidson group exist today?

   a. Over 1,400
   b. Over 1,600
   c. Over 1,800
   d. Over 2,000

ANSWER KEY

1. D: Yonkers, MC

2. C: The Hollister Riot

3. C: Motorcycle Club

4. A: 1%

5. True

6. False

7. False

8. D: Gypsy Tour Rally

9. C: Outlaw

10. False

11. D: Harleys were cheaper than foreign imported motorcycles

12. C: Hell's Angels

13. B: Kuttes (Cuts)

14. True

15. C: One-Eyed Snakes

16. D: Hunter S. Thompson

17. D: One year

18. True

19. C: Harley Owners Group (HOG)

20. A: Over 1,400 chapters

FACTS, FACTOIDS,
AND INTERESTING STORIES

- Harley-Davidson Motor Company has never supported the ideals of the outlaw motorcycle gangs but has been a heavy supporter of law-abiding motorcycle clubs and organizations.
- The founder of Oakland's Hell's Angels chapter, Sonny Berger, once explained that Harley-Davidson motorcycles were popular because they were available, not because they were particularly loyal to the brand.
- The Hell's Angels were hired to work as security to the Altamont Free Concert in 1969. During a performance of the Rolling Stones, a small brawl broke out near the stage.

  o Security moved in quickly and got involved in the fight.
  o An 18-year-old Black man named Meredith Hunter was stabbed and killed during the fight.

- Harley-Davidsons were the choice motorcycles for many of the early motorcycle clubs and gangs because Harleys were cheap, available in surplus (especially after the Second World War), and easy to obtain.
- Harley-Davidson motorcycles became synonymous with liberty, independence, rebellion, virility,

freedom, strength, and power—the ideals embraced by motorcycle clubs, gangs, and organizations.

- Cruisers, a popular model produced by Harley-Davidson, were a go-to choice for many motorcycle clubs due to their comfort, size, low maintenance requirements, versatility, and tough appearance.
- While there are motorcycle clubs that take part in an array of violent and criminal activities, much of this has been sensationalized as a standard occurrence among all motorcycle clubs, which is entirely untrue.
  - Although a fair majority of motorcycle clubs in the world are fraternal organizations and have no connections to any criminal activity, outlaw motorcycle clubs are more well known than the non-gang–related ones.
    - Some illegal activity often associated with outlaw motorcycle gangs includes assault, domestic abuse, weapons trafficking, parole violations, drug possession, intimidation, distribution of stolen motorcycle parts, drug trafficking, weapons possession, gambling, extortion, prostitution, and many other criminal offenses.
- The Hollister Riot is best remembered because of the supposed remarks made by the American Motorcyclist Association (AMA) stating that 99% of the participants of the Gypsy Tour Rally were good,

111

law-abiding, and honest people who did not take part. That left the remaining 1% of the attendees to be the unruly individuals solely responsible for the problems.

- o   This is where the 1% patch, which appears on the attire of specific motorcycle gangs, originates.

  - ▪ These patches were made to distinguish between the non-criminal motorcycle clubs and those that take part in criminal activities.

CHAPTER 11

THE HISTORY OF HARLEY-DAVIDSON IN THE RACING CIRCUIT

TRIVIA TIME

1. Harley-Davidson did not immediately take part in motorcycle racing when it first founded its company in 1903. Instead, after ten years of production, Harley-Davidson created a racing department in 1913.

   a. True
   b. False

2. What was the first sanctioned speed sport in motorcycle racing that Harley-Davidson took part in, which has since become a favorite sport?

   a. Hill climbing
   b. Downhill racing
   c. Cross country racing
   d. Sprint races

3. What was the name of the first competition team formed by the Harley-Davidson Motor Company?

a. Smash Brothers
b. Wrecking Crew
c. Bash Brothers
d. Crash Squad

4. In 1921, Otto Walker set a world record racing a Harley-Davidson at over what speed for the first time?

    a. 75 mph
    b. 80 mph
    c. 90 mph
    d. 100 mph

5. Between 1932 and 1936, who won all of the AMA Grand National Championships?

    a. William Davidson Jr.
    b. Walter G. Davidson
    c. Otto Walker
    d. Joe Petrali

6. Which race did William (Bill) Davidson Jr. win in 1934 with a total of 997 out of a possible 1,000 points?

    a. AMA Grand National Dirt Track Event
    b. Daytona 200
    c. Jackpine Endurance Test
    d. AMA Gypsy Tour Rally

7. What was the record land speed achieved by Joe Petrali in the late 1930s?

    a. 123 mph

b. 128 mph
c. 136 mph
d. 139 mph

8. Which Harley-Davidson did Joe Petrali ride to set this record?

   a. Model D
   b. EL Racer
   c. Model JE
   d. XLH Sportster

9. All motorcycle races are safe.

   a. True
   b. False

10. How many consecutive AMA Grand National Dirt Track Events did legendary racer Jimmy Chan win between 1947 and 1949?

    a. 6
    b. 5
    c. 4
    d. 3

11. Who won the AMA Grand National Championship for Harley-Davidson in 1950 for dirt-track racing, in which Harley-Davidson racers won 18 out of 25 National Championships?

    a. Joe Petrali
    b. Larry Headrick
    c. Scott Parker

d. William Davidson Jr.

12. In which event did Harley-Davidson have eight successive wins between 1954 and 1961?

    a. AMA National Dirt Track Event

    b. Daytona 200

    c. AMA Grand National Series

    d. AMA Motocross Championship

13. Which model of Harley-Davidson has a reputation as one of the best road racing motorcycles?

    a. XR750

    b. Knucklehead

    c. Fat Boy

    d. Street Glide

14. In which race did Brad Andres win first place in 1960, where he and the top 14 finishers all rode 750 KR Harley-Davidsons?

    a. MotoGP

    b. Gypsy Tour Rally

    c. AMA Grand National Championship

    d. Daytona 200

15. Which engine was in the Harley-Davidson that Bart Markel used to win the AMA Grand National Championship in 1965 and 1966?

    a. Flathead

    b. Knucklehead

    c. V-twin

d. Sprint CR

16. What was the average speed of the Sportster XR-750 racer introduced in 1970?

    a. 245 mph
    b. 265 mph
    c. 285 mph
    d. 295 mph

17. No bystander has ever died at a motorcycle-racing event.

    a. True
    b. False

18. Who is thought to be one of the most successful Harley-Davidson racers, first joining the team in 1981?

    a. Randy Goss
    b. Eddie Karwiec
    c. Scott Parker
    d. Kenny Coolbeth

19. How many Grand National Championships did the previously mentioned racer earn over the course of his career?

    a. 6 championships
    b. 7 championships
    c. 8 championships
    d. 9 championships

20. In 2001, who was the first woman to win a national event at the Formula USA National Dirt Track Series and join the Harley-Davidson racing team at 17 years of age?

    a. Jennifer Snyder
    b. Ana Carrasco
    c. Beryl Swain
    d. Olga Kevelos

ANSWER KEY

1. True

2. A: Hill climbing

3. B: Wrecking Crew

4. D: 100 mph

5. D: Joe Petrali

6. C: Jackpine Endurance Test

7. C: 136 mph

8. B: EL Racer

9. False

10. D: 3

11. B: Larry Headrick

12. C: AMA Grand National Series

13. A: XR-750

14. D: Daytona 200

15. D: Sprint CR

16. B: 265 mph

17. False

18. C: Scott Parker

19. D: 9 championships

20. A: Jennifer Snyder

FACTS, FACTOIDS,
AND INTERESTING STORIES

- Racing, on track or on dirt, is one of the most popular activities that riders enjoy taking part in with their Harley-Davidsons and other motorcycles.
- In 1912, at a race in Newark, New Jersey, four spectators, and two racers were killed, including the crashing driver Eddie Hasha. Ten more onlookers were also wounded in the accident.
  - The cause of the accident was attributed to the motordome's board tracks being unstable.
    - The use of boards for the tracks in racing fell out of favor because of this disaster.
- Carroll Resweber won four AMA Grand National Championships during his time as a Harley-Davidson racer, with his winning streak starting in 1958.
- The XR-750 debuted in 1972 and became a premier choice for dirt track racing in the 1970s.
- Dick O'Brien is an AMA legend and was Harley-Davidson's racing director from 1957 to 1983, helping bolster the company's racing department to legendary levels.
- The American Motorcycle Association opened a Motorcycle Hall of Fame in 1990 in Pickerington, Ohio.

- It recognizes the sport of motorcycle racing, famous racers, and the motorcycles themselves.
- It also features motorcycle gear, collectibles, equipment, and clothing.

- Joe Petralli was one of the first salaried "factory racers," acting as a competitor, specifically riding as a representative of the company.
- Harley-Davidson's Wrecking Crew racing team merged with the Factory Team. It included independent racers who were separate but associated with the Harley-Davidson racing squad.
- Jason McRoy, a British downhill mountain bike racer, died in an accident on the A628 in England while riding his Harley-Davidson.
- Harley-Davidson racer Eddie Krawiec won for the Harley-Davidson racing team for the fifth time in 2011.

CHAPTER 12:

HARLEY-DAVIDSON, THE MOTORCYCLE, AND TIMELESS ROCK MUSIC

TRIVIA TIME

1. What was the name of the 1964 Shangri-Las song that told of a tragic love story between a bad-boy biker and a young woman?

   a. "My Guy"
   b. "Don't Throw Your Love Away"
   c. "Leader of the Pack"
   d. "Little Honda"

2. Which band sang the 1968 hit "Born to Be Wild," a classic riding song for motorcyclists?

   a. Led Zeppelin
   b. Cream
   c. The Who
   d. Steppenwolf

3. Which 1968 Arlo Guthrie song off the album *Alice's Restaurant* speaks about the open road, riding fast

motorcycles, and guitars? It famously starts off with the line, "I don't want a pickle/Just want to ride my motorcycle."

    a. "The Motorcycle Song"
    b. "Alice's Restaurant Massacre"
    c. "Last to Leave"
    d. "Highway in the Wind"

4. Which singer wrote and performed the 1971 funk/ rock classic "Ezy Rider"?

    a. Janis Joplin
    b. Paul McCartney
    c. Jimi Hendrix
    d. Carlos Santana

5. The 1970 song "The Long Lonesome Highway" by Michael Parks tells of the freedoms of the open road found while riding on a motorcycle.

    a. True
    b. False

6. Gregg Allman's 1970 song "Midnight Rider" tells of what subject matter pertaining to motorcycle culture that was greatly popularized?

    a. A bad-boy biker and his tragic love story with a good girl
    b. A broke outlaw traveling on a never-ending open road
    c. A couple riding a motorcycle across the country
    d. A man chasing his dreams on the road to Hollywood

7. In the Sailcat song "Motorcycle Mama," what did the singer promise to get for his and his girlfriend's baby so that the three of them could go "see the world through my Harley"?

   a. A little motorcycle
   b. A seatbelt
   c. Leather chaps
   d. A sidecar

8. Which 1970s song tells of a man putting together a "basket case" Harley-Davidson only to have the newly assembled bike break down (a common problem during the AMF era)?

   a. "Take It Easy" by The Eagles
   b. "Harley-Davidson Blues" by Canned Heat
   c. "Truckin'" by Grateful Dead
   d. "My Sharona" by The Knack

9. What kind of motorcycle is described in Bruce Springsteen's 1973 hit "Born to Run"?

   a. Sportster racing bike
   b. Scooter
   c. Motocross bike
   d. Hot Rod Chopper

10. Which outlaw biker gang served as the unofficial bodyguards for Mötorhead frontman Lemmy, and whose outlaw ideal is described in the 1977 song "Iron Horse/Born to Lose"?

   a. The Mongols

b. The Sons of Silence

c. The Hell's Angels

d. The Pagans

11. Which singer describes a disastrous motorcycle crash in the 1979 song "Bat Out of Hell"?

a. Dr. Hook

b. Sting

c. Meat Loaf

d. Elton John

12. The band Saxon sang their ode to the life of a "Motorcycle Man" on which 1980 album?

a. *Wheels of Steel*

b. *Crusader*

c. *Strong Arm of the Law*

d. *Denim and Leather*

13. Which famous Harley-Davidson engine design is featured in a 1982 country-rock song about a man's love for his trusty motorcycle through the years?

a. "On the Road Again" by Willie Nelson

b. "Drive" by The Cars

c. "I Ran (So Far Away)" by A Flock of Seagulls

d. "Panhead Forever" by David Allan Coe

14. Fist fighting and motorcycles are the core values described in the badass 1982 rock song "Bad to the Bone" by George Thorogood and the Destroyers.

a. True

b. False

15. Which set of lyrics can be found in the 1983 song "Ride to Live, Live to Ride" by Twisted Sister?

    a. "Cold steel and hot fuel injected's the dream that fills his brain/But no, not slow, the speed fever grows/He rides/He sees/He knows"
    b. "There's a man in the shadows with a gun in his eye/And a blade shining oh so bright/ There's evil in the air, and there's thunder in the sky"
    c. "He sort of smiled and kissed me goodbye/ The tears were beginning to show/As he drove away on that rainy night"
    d. "I want to guard your dreams, and visions/ Just wrap your legs 'round these velvet rims/ And strap your hands across my engines"

16. What song featured the lyrics "I play for keeps 'cause I might not make it back/I've been everywhere, still I'm standing tall/I've seen a million faces, and I've rocked them all"?

    a. "Sweet Child O' Mine" by Guns N' Roses
    b. "Where the Streets Have No Name" by U2
    c. "Pour Some Sugar on Me" by Def Leppard
    d. "Wanted Dead or Alive" by Bon Jovi

17. Which song by the band Poison captured the ideal of a modern warrior on a horse of chrome in its lyrics?

    a. "Every Rose Has Its Thorn"
    b. "Ride the Wind"
    c. "Life Goes On"
    d. "Talk Dirty to Me"

18. Which 1991 Richard Thompson song tells of a career criminal falling in love and gifting his precious ride to his girlfriend before succumbing to injuries sustained during a robbery gone bad?

    a. "'52 Vincent Black Lightening"
    b. "Dad's Going to Kill Me"
    c. "Keep Your Distance"
    d. "Last Shift"

19. Which band wrote the song "One Last Ride"?

    a. Judas Priest
    b. Lynyrd Skynyrd
    c. Molly Hatchet
    d. Foghat

20. Which song was used as the theme song for *Sons of Anarchy*?

    a. "This Life" by Curtis Stigers and the Forest Rangers
    b. "Motorcycle Man" by Wheels of Steel
    c. "Highway to Hell" by AC/DC
    d. "Sympathy for the Devil" by the Rolling Stones

ANSWER KEY

1. C: "The Leader of the Pack"

2. D: Steppenwolf

3. A: "Motorcycle Song"

4. C: Jimi Hendrix

5. True

6. B: A broke outlaw traveling on a never-ending open road

7. D: A sidecar

8. B: "Harley-Davidson Blues" by Canned Heat

9. D: Hot Rod Chopper

10. C: The Hell's Angels

11. C: Meat Loaf

12. A: Wheels of Steel

13. D: "Panhead Forever" by David Allan Coe

14. False

15. A: "Cold steel and hot fuel injected's the dream that fills his brain/But no, not slow, the speed fever grows/He rides/He sees/He knows"

16. D: "Wanted Dead or Alive" by Bon Jovi

17. B: "Ride the Wind"

18. A: "'52 Vincent Black Lightening"

19. C: Molly Hatchet

20. D: "This Life" by Curtis Stigers and the Forest Rangers

FACTS, FACTOIDS, AND INTERESTING STORIES

- Motorcycle music has influenced a variety of different genres, ranging from punk to heavy metal to classic rock to outlaw country.
- Elvis Presley's last motorcycle was a 1976 Harley-Davidson FLH 1200 Electra Glide.
  - Prior to the auction in 2019, it was predicted to sell for at least two million dollars.
    - When it did go to auction, it was sold for only $800,000.
- Singer Mitch Lucker of the deathcore metal band Suicide Silence died on November 1, 2012, in Huntington, California, from injuries he sustained when he crashed his 2013 Harley-Davidson on Halloween.
- Rock 'n' roll embraced the ideals of the modern-day cowboy, the road warrior, the outlaw, the bad boy, and the leather jacket-wearing members of the motorcycle culture that arose in the 1950s.
- There have been many songs describing outlaw life, especially in country, country rock, outlaw country, and rock 'n' roll songs.
  - There are thousands of songs describing life on a motorcycle or riding a motorcycle.

- The music video for the song "Killed by Death" by Mötorhead shows off a classic Harley-Davidson with Lemmy riding a Harley-Davidson Ironhead Sportster.
- Even when they did not explicitly describe Harley-Davidsons, many rock songs described the chrome, leather, and roaring engines that could only belong to a Harley-Davidson, a beloved American classic.
- Lady Gaga's music video for the song "Judas" features the singer riding on the back of a 2002 Harley Sporter with actor Norman Reedus.
- Duane Allman, elder brother of Gregg Allman and member of the Allman Brothers, died in a motorcycle crash in Macon, Georgia, in October 1971 while riding a Harley-Davidson Sportster.
  - The two brothers' last conversation had been an argument over drugs.
  - Duane Allman had been speeding when a truck stopped in an intersection.
    - He hit the vehicle and was thrown from his bike, which landed on him.
      - He died hours later in the hospital due to the injuries he sustained in the crash.

CHAPTER 13:

CELEBRITY HARLEY-DAVIDSON OWNERS

TRIVIA TIME

1. Which 2014 model Harley-Davidson did Alice Cooper famously give to auction off for charity?

   a. Dyna Wide Glide
   b. Panhead
   c. Bopper
   d. Sportster XL 1200X

2. Which actor/comedian got their start on the show *In Living Color* and rode a custom Harley-Davidson Road King?

   a. Damon Wayans
   b. Jim Carrey
   c. Jamie Foxx
   d. David Alan Grier

3. Who has been dubbed the "Queen of Rock 'n' Roll," got her start with her husband and their band in the late 1950s, became a legendary solo rock vocal icon, appeared in incredibly memorable film roles such as

the Acid Queen in *Tommy* and Aunty Entity in *Mad Max Beyond Thunderdome* and rode a 1993 Harley-Davidson Electra-Glide during the mid-90s?

   a. Tina Turner

   b. Angela Basset

   c. Diana Ross

   d. Grace Slick

4. Despite injuries he had sustained from a motorcycle crash on a Triumph motorcycle in 1966, which model Harley-Davidson did folk-rock legend and Nobel Laureate Bob Dylan acknowledge to be the first motorcycle he rode, initiating his love for quality motorcycles?

   a. Shovelhead

   b. Chopper

   c. Knucklehead

   d. Café Racer

5. Which *Terminator 2* actor currently serves as the president of the motorcycle club "The Boozefighters" and has a history of riding several Harley-Davidson motorcycles throughout his life?

   a. Arnold Schwarzenegger

   b. Joe Morton

   c. Robert Patrick

   d. Edward Furlong

6. Which internationally renowned film superstar and Academy Award winner was in her mid-to-late

fifties when she was gifted a 1988 Harley-Davidson 883 "Hugger" by her dear friend/lover Malcolm Forbes?

   a. Audrey Hepburn
   b. Elizabeth Taylor
   c. Miyoshi Umeki
   d. Shirley MacLaine

7. This rock 'n' roll/pop legend and award-winning actress has owned several Harley-Davidsons and made appearances at rallies, parades, and other Harley-Davidson events.

   a. Stevie Nicks
   b. Janis Joplin
   c. Petula Clark
   d. Cher

8. Collector of many motorcycles — including a Suzuki GSX-R750, 1985 Harley-Davidson Shovelhead, a Norton Commando, and a 2005 Harley-Davidson Dyna Wide Glide — which famous actor got his start in '80s comedies and became a staple in action films throughout the '90s, '00s, and 2010s?

   a. Keanu Reeves
   b. Sean Penn
   c. Robert Downey Jr.
   d. Patrick Swayze

9. What quintessential outlaw country singer is best known to have owned several different motorcycles, including Boppers and Sportsters?

   a. Willie Nelson
   b. Johnny Cash
   c. David Allan Coe
   d. Waylon Jennings

10. Which motorcycle enthusiast (and Harley-Davidson owner) made a name for himself as a comedian and then the host of the *Tonight Show* from the 1990s until 2014?

    a. Johnny Carson
    b. Jay Leno
    c. Conan O'Brien
    d. Jimmy Fallon

11. In the late 2000s, which rapper/actor became an owner of Harley-Davidsons after partnering with Harley-Davidson to auction off bikes to help kids in lower-income areas?

    a. Ice-T
    b. Eminem
    c. Ludacris
    d. Ice Cube

12. Starting off his career as a part of the All-New Mickey Mouse Club and then an international superstar with the boy band NSYNC, Justin Timberlake has a custom

Harley-Davidson he enjoys riding around Los Angeles.

   a. True

   b. False

13. Which actor, known for both his action-thriller films and his romantic roles, is also known for his love of motorcycles but is best remembered for erroneously putting gasoline in his Harley-Davidson Shovelhead's oil tank?

   a. George Clooney

   b. Matt Damon

   c. Ben Affleck

   d. Brad Pitt

14. Which Golden Age film star, also called the "King of Hollywood," owned a 1934 Harley-Davidson 45CI RL?

   a. Cary Grant

   b. Gary Cooper

   c. Gregory Peck

   d. Clark Gable

15. Rapper and actress Queen Latifah is the proud owner of a 1982 Harley-Davidson Knucklehead.

   a. True

   b. False

16. Which former *Saturday Night Live* cast member is known for owning a Harley-Davidson that he enjoys riding wherever he can?

a. Adam Sandler
b. Steve Martin
c. Dan Aykroyd
d. Chevy Chase

17. Which singer, dancer, actress, and model — who made a name for herself from the 1950s into the early 1970s — has been a fan of the Harley-Davidsons for years and famously sang an homage to the motorcycles in the 1968 song "Harley-Davidson"?

a. Brigitte Bardot
b. Doris Day
c. Josephine Baker
d. Connie Francis

18. Which Harley-Davidson enthusiast is also a best-selling horror author?

a. Clive Barker
b. Dean Koontz
c. R.L. Stine
d. Stephen King

19. Which Grammy award-winning pop-rocker owns a Harley Sportster XL Iron 883N and is known for her powerful voice, acrobatic skills, and humor?

a. Christina Aguilera
b. Pink (P!nk)
c. Adele
d. Lady Gaga

20. Which actor, after playing a variety of roles and overcoming drug addiction, is remembered for riding a custom Harley-Davidson Chopper made for a series of exploitation action films?

   a. Sylvester Stallone
   b. Carl Weathers
   c. Danny Trejo
   d. Bruce Willis

ANSWER KEY

1. D: Sportster XL 1200X

2. B: Jim Carrey

3. A: Tina Turner

4. C: Knucklehead

5. C: Robert Patrick

6. B: Elizabeth Taylor

7. D: Cher

8. A: Keanu Reeves

9. C: David Allen Coe

10. B: Jay Leno

11. C: Ludacris

12. True

13. D: Brad Pitt

14. D: Clark Gable

15. False

16. C: Dan Aykroyd

17. A: Bridgette Bardot

18. D: Stephen King

19. B: Pink (P!nk)

20. C: Danny Trejo

FACTS, FACTOIDS, AND INTERESTING STORIES

- Cher owned a 1994 Fat Boy, which she rode until 2003 when she sold it.
- The third person to walk on the moon as a part of the famous Apollo missions, astronaut Pete Conrad (Charles "Pete" Conrad Jr.), died in a hospital from injuries that he sustained in a July 1999 motorcycle crash while traveling with friends and family.
  - He had been riding his 1996 Harley-Davidson in Ojai, California.
  - He had been obeying traffic laws and wearing a helmet at the time of his crash.
  - He died shortly after his crash.
  - Due to his comparatively short stature, he notably said, "That may have been a small one for Neil [Armstrong], but that is a long one for me" in reference to Neil Armstrong's famed statement, "That's one small step for man, one giant leap for mankind."
- Charlie Hunnam, the lead actor from the show *Sons of Anarchy*, rides the same bike that he rode on the show, an early-aughts Harley-Davidson Dyna Super Glide.

- *Saturday Night Live* alum and comedic actor Dan Aykroyd owns a Harley-Davidson Softail and a 2003 Harley-Davidson Police FLHP.

  - Talking about riding on a motorcycle, Aykroyd said, "When you're on the bike, all you're doing is concentrating on staying alive. You get into the rhythm of the road, and it's quite zen."

- Kid Rock is a motorcycle enthusiast with a wide selection of motorcycles, including several Harley-Davidsons.

  - He has a number of Harley-Davidsons of his own, as well as ones he rode for sponsorship.

  - He hosted a summer tour, which was sponsored in 2013-2014 for the company's 110th anniversary.

- Scottish actor Ewan McGregor, famous for his many diverse roles, including Obi-Wan Kenobi in the *Star Wars* prequel trilogy and the upcoming *Obi-Wan* series on Disney+, is a well-known motorcycle enthusiast who has traveled across multiple countries on different motorcycles for different causes, including delivering medicine.

  - One of his more recent trips in 2019 was documented for Apple TV+ and dubbed *The Long Way Up*, where he and his friend Charley Boorman rode Harley-Davidson LiveWire motorcycles from Patagonia, Argentina, to California.

- Lawrence Desmedt, best known as Indian Larry, was a renowned motorcycle builder, designer, stunt rider, and motorcycle enthusiast. He established himself as a traditional builder of choppers in New York City from the 1980s into the 2000s after falling in love with motorcycles as a child.

    o His first motorcycle was a 1939 Knucklehead that he rebuilt from scratch.

    o Indian Larry was killed late in the summer of 2004.

        - While performing a stunt in North Carolina, he fell off his motorcycle and sustained traumatic head injuries.

            - He died of his wounds two days later.

- In the summer of 2002, NASCAR driver Andy Kirby was killed when he crashed his 1985 Harley-Davidson in an accident in his hometown of White House, Tennessee.

- Maroon 5 lead singer and judge on *The Voice*, Adam Levine, is another rock star who rode a Harley-Davidson.

- James Dean, one of the original 1950s rebels and star of *Rebel Without a Cause*, owned several Harley-Davidsons and loved to ride them and his other motorcycles. His collection included a Triumph TR 5 Trophy, a Royal Enfield 500, a Norton 500, and an Indian 500.

- Robert Craig "Evel" Knievel owned a Harley-Davidson XR750 and often performed stunts on his beloved motorcycles.
- Author John Gardner, who wrote several books, including the novel *Grendel*, was killed in a motorcycle accident near his home in Pennsylvania when he lost control of his 1979 Harley, went onto a dirt shoulder, and hit a guard rail.

  - His injuries were primarily caused by blunt force trauma from his body hitting the handlebars.
  - He had been previously drinking (although not at the limit) and was believed to have been exhausted and overworked.
  - His wedding was four days away at the time of his death.

- Elizabeth Taylor's motorcycle was nicknamed "Purple Passion."

  - Michael Forbes, who had given her the bike, was an enthusiastic collector of Harley-Davidsons.

CHAPTER 14:

ACCESSORIES, GEAR, AND PARTS

TRIVIA TIME

1. What is the official name of the Harley-Davidson skull that is a frequent adornment for many customizations, decals, and stylistic designs?

   a. Goode Bone
   b. Davidson Harley
   c. Willie G. Skull
   d. Walter D. Skull

2. What do motorcyclists often call the optional fixture for the passenger backrest that sits at the end of the seat?

   a. "Backboard"
   b. "Back rest"
   c. "Sissy bar"
   d. "Pussy bar"

3. Which attachment became a popular way for a motorcycle to carry an extra passenger?

   a. Sidecar

b. Back car

c. Seat extenders

d. Wider back

4. What was the primary way that Harley-Davidson successfully marketed its products, accessories, and parts throughout the 1900s and into the modern era?

   a. Books

   b. Catalogs

   c. Billboards

   d. Posters

5. Which accessory has been responsible for saving thousands of motorcyclists from severe traumatic brain injuries and death and is one of the most important parts of any motorcyclist's attire?

   a. Face masks

   b. Padded hats

   c. Baseball caps

   d. Helmets

6. What is the most popular item sold bearing the Harley-Davidson name (aside from the motorcycles themselves)?

   a. Shoes

   b. Backpacks

   c. Shirts

   d. Dog bowls

7. Which accessory is both vitally important for a Harley-Davidson owner to fix their motorcycle and an essential purchase for any mechanic?

a. Gloves
b. Tool kits
c. Tire pump
d. Rubber cement

8. All Harley-Davidson models are equipped with windshields and deflectors.

   a. True
   b. False

9. What do they call the metal or plastic pieces that are added to motorcycles, such as the Harley-Davidson KR, to increase streamlining and reduce drag?

   a. Racers
   b. Draggers
   c. Streamliners
   d. Fairings

10. Which accessory is often added to motorcycles along certain ridges and/or parts to enhance the paint job, counter the color of the motorcycles, and decorate it, often appearing in silver, red, black, or gold?

    a. Trim
    b. Rim
    c. Adorns
    d. Borders

11. Windshields are traditionally taller than wind deflectors.

    a. True
    b. False

12. What do motorcyclists frequently call the tall, exaggerated handlebars that are added most commonly to the Chopper models?

    a. Long arms

    b. Chopper drapers

    c. Ape hangers

    d. Handlers

13. Like that of the *Ghost Rider*, what are a popular decoration that is often added to motorcycles to denote "speed" and a tough look?

    a. Stripes

    b. Waves

    c. Stars

    d. Flames

14. What is one of the most popular Harley-Davidson logos that adorn many Harley-Davidson accessories, products, and parts?

    a. Motorcycle wheels

    b. Bar and shield

    c. Handlebars

    d. Diamonds

15. Rather than buy a pre-built or standard motorcycle from a factory, restoring vintage motorcycles is an incredibly popular hobby among many motorcycle enthusiasts.

    a. True

    b. False

16. Which part of a motorcycle engine is frequently featured in many Harley-Davidsons, especially in decals, artwork, logos, and or tattoos for a rough and cool look, often with flames or skulls?

    a. Oil pump
    b. Pushrod
    c. Pistons
    d. Crankshaft

17. Which part of a motorcycle, often featured as an accessory and not as a standard off-the-line production piece, is often installed to shield motorcycle engines and bodyboards (and potentially can protect riders from injuries) if one were to get into an accident?

    a. Engine covers
    b. Crash bars
    c. Sliders
    d. Luggage racks

18. What is the safest way for motorcyclists to travel with luggage or equipment without wearing it on their bodies?

    a. Tail bags
    b. Sidecars
    c. Windshields
    d. Luggage rack

19. Trunks are not a standard feature on most Harley-Davidsons but can be purchased and installed on many models.

a. True

b. False

20. What is another name for saddlebags that are often strapped or installed to the back end of a motorcycle?

    a. Saddlers

    b. Leather bags

    c. Panniers

    d. Tail bags

ANSWER KEY

1. C: Willie G. Skull

2. C: "Sissy Bar"

3. A: Sidecar

4. B: Catalogues

5. D: Helmets

6. C: Shirts

7. B: Tool kits

8. False

9. D: Fairings

10. A: Trim

11. True

12. C: Ape hangers

13. D: Flames

14. B: Bar and shield

15. True

16. C: Pistons

17. B: Crash bars

18. D: Luggage racks

19. True

20. C: Tank bags

FACTS, FACTOIDS, AND INTERESTING STORIES

- Typical Harley-Davidsons come off the production line with standard features, but many Harley-Davidson owners choose to add parts and accessories to enhance their rides and make them unique.
- T-shirts, hats, leathers, backpacks, saddlebags, jewelry, sweatshirts, baby onesies, coffee cups, dog collars, decals, decorative hardware, and motorcycle covers are frequently purchased products for Harley-Davidson fans.
- Customization of motorcycles is incredibly common, ranging from paint jobs to detailing, accessories, or installing new parts to enhance their rides. Upgrades might include radios, trailer hitches, compartments, Bluetooth, and cameras.
- The eagle, skull, and flames are popular symbols that are often associated with Harley-Davidson, along with the bar and shield.

CHAPTER 15:

SUPERSTITION, MISCONCEPTIONS, AND MYTHS OF MOTORCYCLES AND HARLEY-DAVIDSONS

TRIVIA TIME

1. Which patron saint is associated with protecting motorcyclists and travelers from the weather, bad events, and rough elements?

    a. St. Michael
    b. St. Christopher
    c. St. George
    d. St. Gabriel

2. Which color is generally associated with bad luck in the motorcycle community and is not often a color of choice for motorcyclists?

    a. Yellow
    b. Green
    c. Pink
    d. Orange

3. Which item should a Harley owner, or any motorcyclist for that matter, never drop, or they may see their head follow suit?

   a. Gloves
   b. Motorcycle manual
   c. Helmet
   d. Leather jacket

4. What should solo riders never do (according to the more superstitious motorcyclists)?

   a. Travel without leather gloves
   b. Wear gold
   c. Eat before riding
   d. Drive with rear pegs down

5. All motorcycle clubs, gangs, and organizations, especially those who ride Harley-Davidsons, are criminals.

   a. True
   b. False

6. For good karma, according to many motorcyclists, what should another biker do if they see a fellow rider pulled over on the side of the road?

   a. Give them the middle finger
   b. Salute
   c. Pull over to ask if they need help
   d. Do nothing

7. What is another name for the small metal bell, often called a "guardian bell," that is found on the lower part, such as the footrest, of many motorcycles?

    a. "Gremlin bell"
    b. "Demon bell"
    c. "Quasimodo bell"
    d. "Devil's bell"

8. Which country was rumored to have bought Harley-Davidson in 2014?

    a. Germany
    b. Japan
    c. England
    d. Mexico

9. In that rumored sale to a foreign country, which company was speculated to have purchased Harley-Davidson Motor Company?

    a. Royal Enfield
    b. Italika
    c. Münch
    d. Kawasaki

10. What was the original carburetor for Harley-Davidson motorcycles thought to have been constructed from?

    a. A modified fireplace flue
    b. A trolley car air compressor
    c. A tomato can
    d. A burner tray for a steam engine

11. According to many, the HOG moniker given to Harley-Davidson came from a piglet named Johnny that Wrecking Crew member Lawrence Ray Weishaar adopted as an unofficial mascot for the team and not from the Harley Owners Group initials.

    a. True
    b. False

12. While the "Fat Boy" model of Harley-Davidson was thought to have been named after the two atomic bombs dropped on Hiroshima and Nagasaki in 1945 by the U.S. military, what was the actual source of the model's name?

    a. The width of new designs
    b. Reference to a former employee
    c. Derived from the "Fat Bob" model
    d. Nickname given by a competitive company

13. Harley-Davidson was the motorcycle of choice for Marlon Brando's Johnny Strabler and his gang, the Black Rebels Motorcycle Club, in the 1953 film *The Wild One*.

    a. True
    b. False

14. Why do motorcyclists often wear leather when they ride?

    a. Leather is part of the original motorcycle outfit and part of Harley-Davidson's heritage.
    b. Leather looks cool.

c. Leather prevents broken bones.

d. Leather helps protect riders from road rash if they crash.

15. Although the invention of the V-twin engine is frequently and incorrectly attributed to Harley-Davidson, in which year did Gottlieb Daimler develop it?

    a. 1886
    b. 1889
    c. 1903
    d. 1908

16. What is the oldest existing Harley-Davidson club, which was founded in 1927?

    a. Harley Owners Group
    b. Motor Maids
    c. Harley-Davidson Club Prague
    d. Crusaders Motorcycle Club

17. The first Harley-Davidson motorcycle model was built in 1901, two years before Harley-Davidson opened its doors as a company.

    a. True
    b. False

18. What is a myth about Harley-Davidson motorcycles that is more likely attributed to the AMF years of the company when the quality of the bikes was not as high as it had been previously?

a. Harley-Davidson motorcycles always leak oil.

b. They are cheap to buy.

c. The engines blow up when revved.

d. The brakes don't work.

19. All Harley-Davidson motorcycle owners are rebels.

    a. True

    b. False

20. What is a common urban legend about a celebrity's motorcycle?

    a. Cher's motorcycle is worth over $4 million and was sold to Chris Pine.

    b. The Harley-Davidson that John Travolta rode in the 2007 film *Wild Hog* is in the Smithsonian Museum.

    c. Elvis Presley's Harley-Davidson was uncovered in a barn or garage.

    d. The LiveWire featured in *Avengers: Age of Ultron* was sold to a collector for $2 million in 2019.

ANSWER KEY

1. B: Saint Christopher

2. B: Green

3. C: Helmet

4. D: Drive with rear pegs down

5. False

6. C: Pull over to ask if they need help

7. A: "Gremlin bell"

8. B: Japan

9. D: Kawasaki

10. C: A tomato can

11. True

12. C: Derived from the "Fat Bob" model

13. False

14. D: Leather protects riders from road rash if they crash.

15. B: 1889

16. C: Harley-Davidson Club Prague

17. True

18. A: Harley-Davidsons always leak oil.

19. False

20. C: Elvis Presley's Harley-Davidson was uncovered in a barn or garage.

FACTS, FACTOIDS, AND INTERESTING STORIES

- It is bad luck to not pull over on your motorcycle and offer assistance if you see another biker on the side of the road.
- Never drop your helmet!
  - As it goes, if you drop your helmet, your head follows.
  - It is an unproven superstition, but it is always wiser to avoid dropping the helmet anyway.

- A common misconception is that the motorcycles in *The Wild One* were Harley-Davidsons, but interestingly, Brando and his gangs all rode British bikes.
  - Marlon Brando rode his own personal Triumph Thunderbird 650 throughout the movie.

- Riding with the rear pegs down is thought to be bad luck when riding alone. It is said to invite "unwelcome" guests like ghosts or gremlins to ride along.
  - It could also summon a curse.
  - The only exception is when riding in a funeral procession for a fellow biker so that the dead can "ride with the motorcyclist."

- A motorcycle that is painted green is often considered to be incredibly unlucky by traditional American motorcyclists because, originally, all those who rode green motorcycles were killed.
  - American soldiers who acted as envoys during the Second World War were killed while riding their military green motorcycles, which were distinguished from ordinary military bikes.
    - They were frequent targets for snipers, bombs, grenades, and heavy machine gunfire.
  - After the war, many of the Harley-Davidsons were returned to the United States and were cheap and easy to acquire.
    - They were not always in the best condition and could cause accidents.
- The F Head model was not named as a reference to "hey, f*ck head," but instead referring to the shape of the valve ports.
- A common misconception attributed to Harley-Davidson motorcycles is that they continually break down or require constant repairs.
  - During the AMF ownership years, Harley-Davidson bikes often leaked oil.
- Superstitious riders put a "gremlin bell" or a guardian bell on their bikes, which is a small metal bell with the bar and shield Harley-Davidson logo.

- It's meant to ward off evil spirits on the road that could cause the rider to break down on a lonesome highway or crash.
- The myth: If the rider buys the bell for themselves, they will have good fortune on the road; if the bell is bought for them by another person, the luck of the rider will be doubled.

Notes

Going Back to the Basics of Human Health

Avoiding the Fads, the Trends, and the Bold-Faced Lies

Updated, Revised, and Reformatted Edition

Mary Frost, M.A.

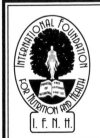

Distributed by the Author and
**INTERNATIONAL FOUNDATION
FOR NUTRITION AND HEALTH**
3963 Mission Blvd.
San Diego, CA 92109
Phone: (858) 488-8932 • FAX: (858) 488-2566
www.ifnh.org • e-mail: ifnh@ifnh.org

Acknowledgements

To Dr. Royal Lee, who was, and still is, a beacon of light for all of us who want to be healthy.

To my husband, Doug, who typed and edited the manuscript I wrote by hand; and who tirelessly supported me though the process of writing this book.

To Dr. Robert Curry, whose support and leadership over the years, has inspired me to keep learning.

To the International Foundation for Nutrition and Health, for carrying the torch of the Lee Foundation, whose initial goal is to educate people on the use of whole food nutrition. To John Brady, III, Director, and all the staff at the Foundation for their many hours of nurturing and unselfish support.

Author's Note

The following principles have guided my writing:

- I don't claim to know everything.
- You and I are always learning.
- This book is in pursuit of the truth.
- This book is a compilation of numerous medical and nutritional studies that I have read and want to share with you.
- You and I are fellow travelers on the road to heath and wellness.

Mary Frost has a B.A. in Journalism from the University of Texas and a Masters of Arts and Liberal Arts from St. Johns College (The Great Books Program). She has been actively involved in health and nutrition for more than 20 years and brings her experience and studies to the forefront as a nutritional journalist.

This book is intended for educational purposes only and should not be used as a guide for diagnosis or treatment of any kind.

Table of Contents

ACKNOWLEDGEMENTS iii

AUTHOR'S NOTE iv

TABLE OF CONTENTS v

INTRODUCTION
Why Whole Food Supplements? vii

CHAPTER 1: OUR HEALTH CRISIS TODAY 1
What To Do? 2
What Is Wrong With This Picture? 3
Where Do We Start? 3
Deforestation 4
Incorrect Farming Methods 8
Fungicides And Pesticides Are Not Working 10
Soil Is A Living Substance 12
How Does A Plant Protect Itself? 13
The Importance Of Trace Minerals 14
Let's Get Real 15
The Chemicalization Of Foods 16
A Dark Period For The FDA Begins 19
The Persecution Of Dr. Lee 20
A Word Or Two About Oils 24
Poisons Found In Refined Oils 25
Water — The Crucial Commodity 26

CHAPTER 2: SYNTHETIC VITAMINS VS. FOOD 29
Why Natural Food Complexes Faded From View 31
Just What Are Natural Complexes? 32
Rats And The RDAs (Recommended Daily
Allowances) 35

Getting To The Core Of The Matter 36
Whole Natural Vitamins vs. Synthetic 37
Potency Is Not Milligrams Or Micrograms Or Units 39
Synthetics Are Not As Effective 40
Antioxidants — The Controversy 42
Antioxidants As A Fad 43
Fads, Trends And Bold-Faced Lies 44
Why Do I Need Vitamins And Minerals If
    I'm Eating Well? 45
A Word About Standard Process 50
The Work In Nutrition Has Already Been Done 53
A Sobering Word 54

CHAPTER 3: FATS, PROTEINS, AND YOUR HEALTH 55
Ancient Civilizations And Low Fat Diets 55
What's Happening Here? 57
Which Way Is Your Metabolism Going? 58
Dieting Is Failing 59
More Than Just Fat 60
High Blood Pressure 60
Enter Cholesterol 62
Diabetes 64
Heart Disease 65
Don't Forget The Eicosanoids 66
A Doctor's View 68

CHAPTER 4: OUR HEALTH 71
Look In The Mirror 72
Digestion vs. Indigestion 73
Summing Up 75
How Do We Find The Answers To Our
    Health Problems? 77
Action Steps To Function Optimally 81

APPENDIX
Footnotes 85
Suggested Reading 90
Index 91

Introduction

Why Whole Food Supplements?

Most of us have gotten used to reading literature proclaiming the benefits of vitamins, deciding what is wrong with us, and heading to the health food store to buy what we have decided we need. Often, we end up buying all kinds of supplements and we are still not any healthier.

I, too, was once a health food store junkie. I had also tried different health professionals with no result. Finally, I found a health professional who determined the underlying cause of my health problem. I was suffering from frequent sinus infections (seven in two years) that always resulted in laryngitis. I took vitamin A (25,000 IU), vitamin E (400 IU), ascorbic acid with rose hips (3,000 mg.), Kyolic garlic, echinacea, golden seal, and homeopathics, and they did not help. Truthfully, I was afraid that my immune system was weakening, and I had visions of dying of pneumonia.

Fortunately, the astute health professional started me on whole food supplements from a company called Standard Process. This company has owned and operated its own organic farms since 1929. Using its whole food supplements, I do not get sick anymore. Now, if I start to get the sniffles, I take some whole food supplements and I am quickly over them. Before, I would take the protocol of the products that I purchased from the health food store, and I would still get sick. I could not prevent it.

What I have come to realize, over the years, is that we cannot understand what any company offers in the way of nutri-

tional supplements unless we understand what has happened, step-by-step, to our food supply. And, we cannot understand what a whole food supplement is unless we understand what most vitamins today really are, which are synthetic. This means that the vitamin B you just picked up in your average health food store or drugstore is derived from coal tar. It is easy to say it is "natural," because it once was — about 150 million years ago — but I like my vegetables a little fresher than that, and I know my body does too. So be aware when synthetic vitamins are promoted as "pure" vitamins.

For years, Americans have gotten used to the "new and improved" idea. We don't even know what the truth is. We don't know how to step back and evaluate whether the information being advertised is a fad or not. We are told not to eat butter, to eat margarine instead. Then, 20 years later, we are told that margarine contains transfats and is dangerous for us. We are told not to eat eggs or beef because they can cause cholesterol problems; then, years later, we are told that they are okay.

So, we are presented with "new medical facts" that are advertised to persuade us to change our eating habits and go in a different direction. What we are getting is what Ralph Nader calls "pseudo-science." And what we are getting are genetically-engineered foods, faulty infomercial health tips, incorrect information about what we are already eating, and tricky nutritional labels that we have no way of deciphering.

We need to stop listening to whom Dr. Bernard Jensen and Mark Anderson refer in their book, *Empty Harvest*, as "those television advertising managers practicing medicine without a brain." *Going Back to the Basics of Human Health* is an attempt to pull back the camouflage and look at the inner workings of this gigantic mess. This book will show why we must tune out the antacid and the low-fat diet food commercials, and why we must watch out for synthetic vitamins, either by themselves or hidden in an herbal formula. It is a guide to know

how to evaluate all of this confusing information and stay healthy.

Standard Process (the manufacturer of the whole food supplements I use) has always made its products available only through health professionals. If you are used to reading labels, the labels on whole food supplements don't look anything like those on synthetic vitamin bottles. The sources are completely different, so the dosage is lower. But, after a while of taking the specific whole food supplements they were evaluated for, most people are amazed at the improvement in their health and want to know more.

In the years that I have been using whole food supplements, I have seen amazing results with all kinds of problems that people present to me. The therapeutic use of whole food supplements, such as those from Standard Process, really help to build the immune system and make people stronger and healthier.

But taking whole food supplements wasn't all that I needed, because eating a low-fat diet had me tired and fatigued most of the time and I couldn't figure it out. Someone introduced me to Jay Robb's *Fat Burning Diet,* and, within a short time, I felt my life-force coming back. It was then that I realized the importance of blood sugar and optimal health. I read everything I could get my hands on, including Dr. Robert Atkins' *New Diet Revolution.* But, it was the book, *Protein Power,* that really opened my eyes. This book leaves no stone unturned in exposing the deadly issue of excessive insulin in the body.

I hope you enjoy reading this information, and that it opens your eyes to what the real issues of health are today in America. The process of gathering this information opened my eyes and changed my life forever.

Going Back to the Basics of Human Health

Avoiding the Fads, the Trends, and the Bold-Faced Lies

1/**Our Health Crisis Today**

"Thus, we should be aware of clinging to vulgar opinions and judge things by reason's way, not by popular say."

—*Montaigne* (1533-1592)

Today Americans are in a health crisis. Is this what we spend our lives working for?

- Three out of every four Americans will get heart disease — two out of every four will die from it. Two hundred thousand Americans die yearly from high blood pressure and strokes.
- According to the American Diabetes Association, the number of diabetics has increased from six to 16 million in the last 15 years. Each day, approximately 2,200 people are diagnosed with Type 2 diabetes in the United States. In 2004, the United Nations and the World Health Organization predicted that the number of cases of Type 2 diabetes will soar from 117 million to 370 million by 2030.
- Roughly 25% of all adult Americans are obese. The Center for Disease Control has called obesity an epidemic, killing almost 500,000 people a year.
- The Merck Manual 2000 cites the number-one cause of death in the world today as malnutrition, with results of immune deficiency and infection.
- According to the PBS program Critical Condition, which delved into the state of America's health care, more than 100 million Americans are chronically ill.
- Some form of depression, anxiety, or fatigue affects over 50% of the population.

These statistics alone are enough to depress you. But, if figures alone don't bring it home, think about it this way: If you filled a Boeing 747 jumbo jet to capacity (300 persons) and computed into airline crashes the number of deaths resulting from heart disease, hypertension and diabetes, you would have 3,650 jumbo jet crashes a year. That would be 10 jumbo jets falling out of the sky every day. How many of us would fly again with such risks involved? It is pretty sick thinking, but it helps to create what scholars have named the "outrage" factor — how people react differently to death or disability from a specific cause.

And, outraged is what we as a nation should be. But we are more concerned when a plane crashes because of the publicity than we are of the number of people dying from heart disease every year. Yet, there is a lot of human misery reflected in these frightening statistics, plus billions of dollars involved in the health care needs these people require. Orthodox medical care spending is now estimated at $1.6 trillion per year. (When I first published this book in 1997, orthodox medical spending was $200 billion per year. That is an increase of eight times the amount of spending in just seven years.) With the average increase in healthcare costs being in double digits every year, can we afford to bury our heads in the sand anymore?

What To Do?

In the attempt to protect themselves and their families from these frightening and serious health problems, Americans are changing their diets and are taking herbs and supplements. One in three Americans seeks alternative treatment, at a cost of $17 billion annually. Over-the-counter vitamin sales are at $6 billion per year. This means that most people pull their vitamins off a shelf with the help of a store clerk. And yet, people are getting sicker. They pump vitamins and eat "right," but that does not seem to be the answer. They are still fatigued, still overweight,

still fighting the cholesterol battle, etc.

Nearly every week most people get at least two or three mailers touting some "new medical cure" or "amazing discoveries." It was in response to this deluge of material that I have been urged to write this book — to enable people to wade through all this information and make informed decisions. There *is* an answer.

What Is Wrong With This Picture?

When people are trying so hard to do the right thing, why aren't the results long-term? Why do they feel so great when they start taking vitamins and later feel fatigued again? Why are 95% of the people who lose weight unable to keep it off? Why are the statistics on heart disease, hypertension, and diabetes getting worse?

My studies have led me to conclude that the three major culprits are:

1. The harm that is done to our food before it even gets to us. The depletion and demineralization of America's topsoil, the contamination of produce by excessive use of pesticides and fungicides, the chemicalization of food through over-processing, enriching, preserving, and the contamination of water through fluoridation.
2. Synthetic vitamins taken as supplements.
3. Low-fat, low-protein, high-carbohydrate diets.

Where Do We Start?

Foods are not what they seem anymore. Consider these facts:

- To get the iron that was available in one cup of spinach in 1945, you would have to consume 65 cups today.
- An orange that contained 50 mg. of natural vitamin C complex in 1950 now contains 5 mg.

3

In most instances, that lovely green salad on your table is practically dead nutritionally.

"We are producing less nutritious food at the highest cost in history while United States farmers are going bankrupt." [1]

How can this be? American's topsoil has been depleted through:

1. Deforestation
2. Incorrect farming methods
3. Overuse of fungicides and pesticides

Deforestation

Deforestation, while not in itself responsible for our nutritionally-dead foods, marks the first major assault in the dismantling of our natural eco-system. The cutting down of massive amounts of trees "laid bare" a disrespect for Mother Nature and a lack of interest in Her inner workings that paved the way for our lack of health today.

When settlers began arriving in America in the 16th century, they found a land in pristine condition. After *thousands* of years of use by Native Americans, the water was still pure. The land was so fertile that if you dropped a seed, it would grow. Trees and forests were everywhere. In fact, in the Iroquois Nation folklore, they would speak of how a squirrel could hop from tree to tree from the Atlantic Ocean to the Mississippi River. When they gave directions, "grandfather trees" were used as landmarks.

Today we are lucky to have any pure water, topsoil, or forests at all. According to the U.S. Environmental Protection Agency in 1990, agricultural pollutants contaminate nearly half the wells and all of the surface streams in this country.

As for topsoil, in Iowa, topsoils that were once a foot deep are today less than six inches deep. Although it doesn't sound like much, six inches can be devastating. The United States Department of Agriculture estimates that a six-inch loss of topsoil, such

as the current one in southern Piedmont, is capable of reducing crop yields by 40% per year." [2]

The European settlers of this country found 18 to 25 inches of rich topsoil in the 1700s. Nowadays, most farmlands are like those in Iowa. In fact, the dust storms that occurred in the 1930s in Kansas that left topsoil on desktops in Washington D.C. are about to return. Statistics say that in 1977, five million acres were severely eroded by wind; and by 1988, estimates were at 25 million acres. (Areas double the size of Maryland and Massachusetts combined.)

"Kansas Congressman Dan Glickman (former head of the USDA) stated in March of 1989, 'It's no secret the central part of America is blowing away right now.'" [3]

The natural trees, grasses, and vegetation that once anchored the soil are gone. To date, over 260 million acres of trees in America have been cut to make way for raising livestock. Trees shade the soil, hold the soil in place, and act as pumps to draw water up near the surface of the ground, thus keeping water tables high. Without trees, the soil gets baked dry by the sun, and eventually gets blown away by the wind or wasted away by rains. West Texas was once covered with tall grasses; now it is a flat, barren area where high winds carrying loose soil can turn the sky black. Over-grazing of cattle pulled these grasses out of the soil, leaving nothing to hold it in place.

When you see pictures in magazines and on television of starving people in East Africa, what you are really seeing is famine caused by a land laid bare through deforestation. In Ethiopia, for example, 90% of the land was covered by forests in 1890 — now barely 5% remains. Environmentalists, realizing this, have tried to stop the current destruction of the Brazilian rain forests, but the massive cutting down of trees continues. America's national parks, our last forest reserves, are being threatened today by adjacent mining activities, clear-cutting, oil and gas exploration, and many other related activities.

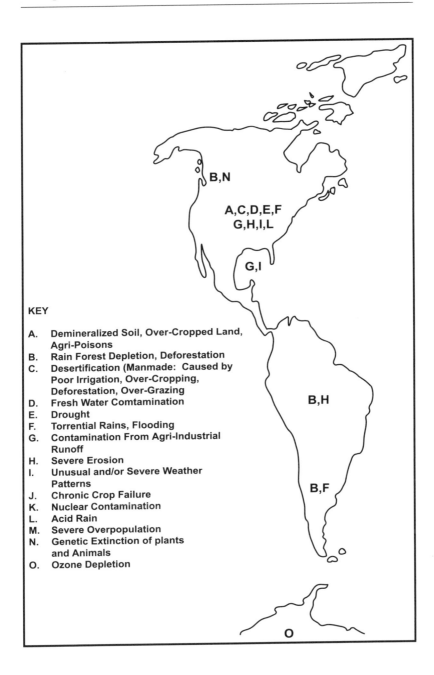

KEY

A. Demineralized Soil, Over-Cropped Land, Agri-Poisons
B. Rain Forest Depletion, Deforestation
C. Desertification (Manmade: Caused by Poor Irrigation, Over-Cropping, Deforestation, Over-Grazing
D. Fresh Water Comtamination
E. Drought
F. Torrential Rains, Flooding
G. Contamination From Agri-Industrial Runoff
H. Severe Erosion
I. Unusual and/or Severe Weather Patterns
J. Chronic Crop Failure
K. Nuclear Contamination
L. Acid Rain
M. Severe Overpopulation
N. Genetic Extinction of plants and Animals
O. Ozone Depletion

B,N

A,C,D,E,F
G,H,I,L

G,I

B,H

B,F

O

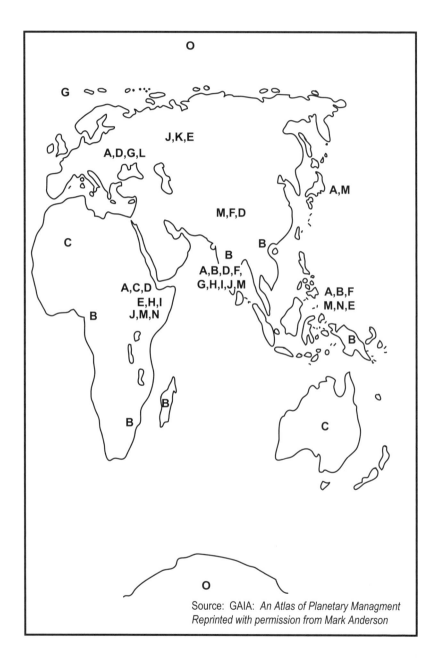

Source: GAIA: *An Atlas of Planetary Managment*
Reprinted with permission from Mark Anderson

Incorrect Farming Methods

The massive use of chemical fertilizers, which are manufactured and shipped around the world by the millions of tons per year, has come to be an accepted method of forcing plants to grow. This method was conceived in a paper published in 1855 by the renowned German chemist, Baron Justus von Liebig. In this document, von Liebig determined that the only minerals plants needed were nitrogen, phosphorous and potassium.

The German chemical industry flourished on this premise, and aggressively marketed it to farmers. The imbalance in trace minerals, fungus and microbial life that this "artificial manure" created was later regretted by von Liebig. At the end of his life, he wrote, "Nature herself points … out to man the proper course of proceeding for keeping up the productiveness of the land." [4]

Some 20 years later, after von Liebig's death, the famed German naturalist, Julius Hensel, ridiculed this nitrogen-phosphorous-potassium theory and encouraged farmers to spread a finely crushed, mineral-rich rock dust on their land. "Those who did were amazed at the quality, strength, and drought resistancy of their crops." [5]

The thriving chemical industrialists were so vicious and vigorous in their attempt to discredit Hensel that his book could not be found anywhere for many years. Their high-handed techniques illustrate how an idea that went against economic interests of the time could be squelched with such ferocity that the farmers were led to conclude that it was false. (Out of sight, out of mind.)

In 1940, Sir Albert Howard published his landmark book, *An Agricultural Testament*. In it, he promoted Hensel's rock dust theories and gave a sobering warning about the use of chemical fertilizers. "The principle followed, based on the von Liebig tradition, is that any deficiencies in the soil can be made up by the addition of suitable chemicals (man-made). This is based on a complete misconception of plant nutrition. It is superficial

and fundamentally unsound. It takes no account of the life of the soil, including mycorrhizal association – the living fungus bridge which connects the soil and sap. Artificial manures lead inevitably to artificial nutrition, artificial food, artificial animals, and finally, to artificial men and women." [6] You can't patent rock dust or manure. You can't patent nature and make immense profits from it.

Chemical fertilizers kill most of the micro-organisms and worms in the topsoil, and then they trickle down through the ground to contaminate underground water supplies. These chemical fertilizers also deplete trace minerals from the soil and contaminate crops. In 1989, the Nutrient Testing Laboratory (NTL) ran mineral analysis tests on commercial produce from regions around the United States. While some foods contained *no* amounts of important minerals such as boron and zinc, all 11 foods tested contained high levels of sodium. The NTL then compared this to the famous H.J. Heinz Nutrition Chart of 1949 and found that sodium content had increased significantly over the last 40 years because artificial chemical fertilizers are either highly concentrated inorganic salts or contain large amounts of inorganic salts.

Most people get confused in the debate between using inorganic or organic fertilizers because they are told most plants absorb inorganic forms of plant nutrients. Organic nutrients must be converted to inorganic forms to become available to the growing plant. So, let's just skip a step, right? Wrong. The slow-release effect of an organic fertilizer is a result of microorganisms in the soil breaking down the organic material into an inorganic form. This process makes the nutrients available for a longer time over the growing season and preserves soil nutrients, instead of leeching them out like chemical fertilizers do.

The oversupply of a chemical form of nitrogen can lead to lush, succulent tissue growth, which is more vulnerable to fungal and bacterial assault, actually more appealing to some insects,

and more prone to injury from heat, cold, or drought — a perfect situation in which to sell *more* pesticides and fungicides.

And what about environmental impact? Almost half of the commercial fertilizers are made from ammonia, which is extracted from natural gas using a complex chemical process. This chemical process releases much carbon dioxide into the atmosphere, which is the main gas responsible for global warming.

Fungicides And Pesticides Are Not Working

Farming has become a high-tech industry, combining technology and economics to exploit the land they farm for profit. "The result: Modern agriculture reduces the role of soil to a substance of convenient texture that holds plants in the vertical position while chemicals are forced up their shaft. Plants stand in the field and receive a chemical enema." [7] (How would you like this?)

The modern corporate farmer looks down from the air-conditioned cab of his $100,000 John Deere tractor and asks, "'What's this?' He sees a little fungus growing on the plant and he says, 'We aren't going to put up with this. We know how to deal with the likes of you!'

He gets into his pickup truck, heads down to the agriculture chemical supply station, and returns loaded with barrels of chemosterilants, with skull and crossbones on their labels. Now he is ready to treat the plant. In the back of his pickup truck are barrels with labels that say things like: 'Use extreme caution — Do not inhale — Use in well-ventilated areas — Do not allow any contact with skin and hair — Do not dispose near water — Keep away from livestock and feed — May cause blindness or death if taken internally — Read all instructions carefully — Federal law requires application in accordance with label data,' and he thinks, "This looks good. Let's apply this to our growing food." [8] Thank goodness for the rise in organic farming and the increase in the numbers of local farmers who actually touch the earth, work with

the soil, and avoid using toxic chemicals on their crops.

Land that once was fertile in the Mississippi Delta is so devoid of worms (a sign of healthy soil) and other microbiotic life, that the remains of harvested crops cannot be turned under any more. This degradation is due to so many years of soil sterilization that the soil is now incapable of even rotting and composting.

According to Professor David Pimental, Department of Entomology at Cornell University, pesticide production from 1945 to 1990 has increased *3,300%.* In the same time period, crop loss due to insects has increased 20%. Pesticides are failing — miserably. (See my website, www.theperfectcrime.com, for more details.)

Pesticides are so deadly that one form, *Zyclan B™,* was used by the Nazis to gas millions of their victims in the concentration camps from 1939 to 1945. Another, *Methyl Isocyanate,* caused the death of over 3,500 people in Bhopal, India, and maimed 200,000 more.

Now the oceans are being ruined by the runoff of chemical fertilizers, pesticides, and animal waste. All areas of the earth's oceans have always contained a wide variety of life. However, there are now areas known as "dead zones," where the oxygen levels are so low that no marine life can live in them. According to OCEANA, one such "dead zone" from the toxic runoff of the Mississippi River forms in the Gulf of Mexico each spring and summer and covers almost 8,000 square miles, or the size of the state of Massachusetts.

Pesticides are difficult to eliminate. Pesticide residues can be found in plants grown in soil previously sprayed years before. In fact, organic farmers in California deal with "Certified Organic" labeling as follows: "No chemical fertilizers or pesticides/fungicides can be used on the land for three years, and the land is built-up organically. At the end of those three years, the produce is tested for pesticide residue. If there is any residue, the farmer must wait another year and have his produce tested again before he can label it "Certified Organic."

You would think that the failure of pesticides to eliminate crop damage would cause these chemical companies to look at possibly contributing to a natural solution. Not so. *Mother Jones*, in its Jan/Feb 1997 issue, published an article called "The Future of Food." Potato and corn seeds are now genetically altered to have a built-in pesticide. Soybean seeds are genetically manipulated to survive direct applications of Roundup™ (so the manufacturer can sell more). These chemical companies are on a destructive track. The article did ask an important question: "Is anyone protecting the consumers?"

An article in *New Yorker* magazine (April 10, 2000) traced the spread of genetically-modified crops this way: "A decade ago, no transgenic crops were commercially available anywhere on earth; in 1995 four million acres had been planted; by 1999, that number had grown to one hundred million. In the United States, half of the enormous soybean crop and more than a third of the corn are products of biotechnology." [9]

That lovely red juicy tomato that came out of your grand-mother's garden full of vitamins, minerals, and enzymes has now been replaced through the "wonders" of bioengineering with a round, faded-red rubbery substance that looks like a tomato. This bioengineering miracle allows it to be harvested by machine and has brought the vitamin C content alone down from 125-150 mg. to 5-0. These rubbery tomato facsimiles contain as few enzymes as possible so they won't bruise or spoil. The enzymes that grandmother's tomatoes had that helped the natural digestion of that tomato are now nonexistent. What a great opportunity for heartburn and an antacid manufacturer. (For more information about biotech, see my website, www.theperfectcrime.com.)

Soil Is A Living Substance

Soil is the basis of all life. The plants that grow in soil are at the lowest end of the food chain and they in turn become food

for animals at the next level of the food chain. These animals are then the food supply for humans at the highest end of the chain.

William Albrecht, PhD, of the University of Missouri, found that he could cure a disease, undulant fever, in livestock and humans by adding trace minerals to the soil in which their food was grown (Henry Ford's only son, Edsel, died from undulant fever.). Albrecht's studies in the 1950s proved beyond a doubt that plants can look and appear healthy but have much lower quantities of nutrients. He also proved that a healthy plant is its own protection against insects, thus eliminating the need for pesticides.

Good soil is composed of 45% minerals and millions of microorganisms. Dr. Albrecht and Dr. Royal Lee, founder of Standard Process, were adamant about this: "When we see a symptom in the plant, it will always correlate to a poison or deficiency in the soil; when we see a disease in the human, it will relate to a poison or deficiency in the food." [10]

Mineral-deficient soil is targeted as one of the original sources of disease in the world today. "Simply stated, food crops grown on depleted soil produce malnourished bodies, and disease preys on malnourished bodies." [11]

How Does A Plant Protect Itself?

What high-tech farmers are lacking is true understanding of the plant's immune system. At the root system, little offshoots called rootlets have hair-like fungi, called *mycorrhiza*, growing on them.

Mineral-rich soil consists of millions of living micro-organisms. Their primary functions are to decompose anything that falls on the land and to break down mineral deposits into plant food. The plant doesn't get devoured by these organisms (bacteria) because the *mycorrhiza* secretes antibiotics to protect the plant. (Keep in mind that penicillin comes from a fungus.)

Nature gave fungi and bacteria an interesting relationship.

They are natural antagonists. They keep each other in check through their competition … the plant, thus protected, is free to absorb the minerals that soil microbial life has released without fear of infection from soil-borne bacteria." [12]

If you see a fungus growing on a plant, it is a self-produced fungus because there was something inferior about the quality of the plant. Nature grows fungus on the inferior plant, and then it dies, decomposes, and begins again — until it gets it right.

The Importance Of Trace Minerals

"Human bodies require nutrition found in the form of plants, meat, milk and eggs." [13]

Since animals get their food directly or indirectly from plants, and plants get their food from the soil, there is a direct link from the soil to human health.

Much is now said in the news media of the importance of different trace minerals, such as selenium, boron, chromium, etc. But just the absence of one trace mineral can cause great health problems.

- Without the trace mineral cobalt, the human body cannot manufacture vitamin B_{12}.
- Without potassium, the heart muscle can be harmed, and the result can be a racing of the heartbeat or tachycardia.
- Without zinc, selenium, sulfur and iron, the liver would be sluggish and/or weak in its abilities to repair damaged tissue, fight infection and detoxify the blood and the bowel.

Remember, plants do not manufacture trace minerals, they *absorb* them. The health of the soil's microbial life depends upon the trace minerals in the soil, and so do *enzymes,* the most important ingredient in plant, animal and human biochemistry. All metabolic processes at every level depend on enzymes. Often, enzymes vital to our immune systems need the rarest trace minerals in order to function. There are 92 known trace elements.

As research continues, it is reasonable to assume that the role of every mineral will be discovered.

Let's Get Real

As we drive in our air-conditioned cars to our air-conditioned offices and sit down in front of our computers — only to go home at night and sit in front of the TV — we are prey to an assault of information unparalleled in history. Yet, so much of what we hear does not take total, factual information into account.

The advocates of whole foods and organic farming are so out-talked by advocates of big business that we can hardly hear the truth through all of their blaring. But our bodies know what is happening. The innate intelligence in our bodies is telling us through heart disease, cancer, AIDS, diabetes, and obesity that something is amiss. And our souls are telling us that profits aren't everything.

"Although the popular ecology movement grabs an occasional headline, what our political leaders, scientists and doctors are unwilling to come to grips with is that we are on the threshold of vast human annihilation. The effect to revitalize the human immune system must begin with a massive effort to return vitality and fertility to our soils." [14]

Consider what historian V.G. Simkovich had to say about the ruins of ancient civilizations: "Look at the unpopulated valleys, at the dead and buried cities, and you can decipher there the promise and the prophecy of us ... Depleted of humus by constant cropping, land could no longer reward labor and support life, so the people abandoned it. Deserted, it became a desert; the light soil was washed by the rain and blown around by the shifting winds." [15]

There is a possibility to reverse this trend. John D. Hamaker, in his monumental work, *The Survival of Civilization*, gives us some guidelines. Hamaker believes that "an all-out global effort

to remineralize the Earth's soils (with rock dust) and the planting of billions of trees, coupled with the elimination of fossil fuel burning, and the development of alternative sources of power (for example, hydrogen, solar and wind) can restore the carbon balance between the land and atmosphere." [16]

The Chemicalization Of Foods

So, we have chopped down millions of acres of trees, over-grazed millions of acres of natural vegetation, poured chemical fertilizers on the soil, and sprayed the plants with fungicides and pesticides. Now, the stage is set to really attack our food supply in earnest. Since whole, natural foods tend to decay or go rancid quickly, methods for producing a long shelf life went into high gear.

When we walk through a grocery store and read labels, many people have never noticed that it really is a journey through a *chemical laboratory*. All the contents have preservatives, additives and synthetic vitamins that we have just come to take for granted. The shocking truth of how all these substances came to be in our foods is not fully understood, but should be.

As Dr. Bernard Jensen and Mark Anderson pointed out in *Empty Harvest*, within a generation following World War I, the foods of commerce took over. "The food supply became bleached, refined, chemically preserved, pasteurized, sterilized, homogenized, hydrogenated, artificially colored, defibered, highly sugared, highly salted, synthetically fortified (enriched), canned, and generally exposed to hundreds of new man-made chemicals." [17]

How did this happen? Where was the Food and Drug Administration (FDA)? The Pure Food and Drug Law was subverted and manipulated by commercial interests starting in 1912. At that time, commercial interests forced Dr. Harvey W. Wiley from his office as founder and head of the Bureau of Chemistry,

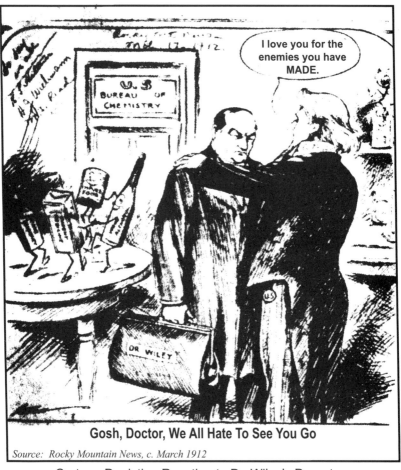

Gosh, Doctor, We All Hate To See You Go

Source: Rocky Mountain News, c. March 1912

Cartoon Depicting Reaction to Dr. Wiley's Departure
from the Bureau of Chemistry

Above, as Dr. Wiley prepares to leave, you will see on the table behind him, caricatures of impure foods, patent medicines, and ersatz substances holding hands holding hands and dancing for joy. In the foreground, Uncle Sam bids farewell and laments the end of Dr. Wiley's career at the Bureau of Chemistry

Photo and caption by permission of Mark Anderson

now known as the FDA. As you can see from the cartoon on the previous page, Dr. Wiley's departure was seen as an open frolic for the synthetic food enhancers.

Before he resigned, Dr. Wiley had ordered the seizure of a shipment of bleached flour because the bleaching process left nitrite residue in the flour. The case of U.S. vs. Lexington Mill and Elevator Company went all the way to the Supreme Court, which ruled in favor of the government and ordered the flour to be destroyed. This decision was then *ignored* by the Department of Agriculture. Dr. Wiley's comment on this was that "so far as bleaching flour is concerned by any process whatever, the Food and Drugs Act does not exist...The very law that the Supreme Court has said was enacted to chiefly protect the public health has been turned into a measure to threaten public health and defraud the purchaser." [18]

When he had filed suit against Coca-Cola™ to keep this artificial product off the market and prohibit its interstate transport, Dr. Wiley said:

"No food product in our country would have any trace of benzoic acid, sulfurous acid or sulfites or any alum or saccharin, save for medical purposes. No soft drink would contain caffeine or theobromine. No bleached flour would enter interstate commerce. Our foods and drugs would be wholly without any form of adulteration and misbranding. The health of our people would be vastly improved and the life greatly extended. The manufacturers of our food supply, and especially the millers, would devote their energies to improving the public health and promoting happiness in every home by the production of whole ground, unbolted cereal flours and meals." [19] (*unbolted* means that the flour is not sifted, therefore the wheat germ is not lost.)

A Dark Period For The FDA Begins

Dr. Wiley's departure led the way for a replacement in the form of Dr. Elmer M. Nelson, a commercially-backed man placed in the front line of all decision making.

The following is an amazing quote from Dr. Nelson's testimony given in federal court to block health food manufacturers from comparing the quality of their products to their synthetic, processed counterparts:

"It is wholly unscientific to state that a well-fed body is more able to resist disease than a less well-fed body. My overall opinion is that there hasn't been enough experimentation to prove dietary deficiencies make one more susceptible to disease." [20]

Unbelievable? Incredible? Is this true science? How many people today know that dietary deficiencies can lead to degenerative diseases, infectious diseases, and functional diseases? The American public has been the official testing "lab" for this kind of fallacious thinking, and it was this kind of reasoning that Dr. Nelson and his team of "experts" expounded for over 10 years in court to get the okay on the synthetics that we have in foods today. It was these courtroom scenes, far way from the public eye, that set the stage for ruined, devitalized food to dominate the marketplace.

It is important to note that landmark works in nutrition by Dr. Weston Price, Dr. Francis Pottenger, Dr. Roger Williams, Dr. Agnes Fay Morgan and Dr. Royal Lee were totally ignored and treated with disdain.

Also ignored was this statement from *Food & Life: The United States Department of Agriculture Yearbook for 1939*: "The chief fault of many American diets is that they provide too little of the essential minerals and vitamins. This fault is due in large measure to the fact that refined foods are consumed in such amounts that the intake of mineral and vitamin-rich foods is lower than it should be." (This booklet is available from www.ifnh.org)

The truth was helpless in the face of an FDA that had unlimited taxpayer dollars at its disposal to promote the commercial interests of the time. We need to understand that the United States government has been controlled by special interests, like the commercial food industry, for nearly 80 years, and people today are just beginning to realize the dangers of this.

The Persecution Of Dr. Lee

Dr. Royal Lee, founder of Standard Process, was a pioneer in the field of nutrition. His cold processing techniques to capture and preserve the nutrients of foods grown on his organic farms are unique even today in the whole food supplement industry. Dr. Lee was concerned about the commercial interests' impact on people's health, especially since these interests gave people *incorrect* information about their foods.

This incorrect information led people to lose sight of the truth. As Dr. Bernard Jensen and Mark Anderson pointed out, "We must not assume that science and truth march straight ahead and that the present is the beneficiary of the accumulated knowledge of the past. Because, in many instances — and health and nutrition is one — the past is full of deception and factual manipulation resulting in the inheritance of a tarnished view of scientific progress." [21]

Dr. Lee's genius as an inventor led to more than 100 patents. He invented the first constant-speed dental drill and one of the first governors for electric motors. He also invented the Endocardiograph (known today as The Acoustic CardioGraph), which helped him develop many of his nutritional formulas. He was a co-inventor for the Norton bombsite during World War II. At the end of the war, he was reported to be worth over $100 million. Dr. Lee later assisted NASA with his motor control design for their Lunar Guidance Systems. However, Dr. Lee's overwhelming passion was nutrition.

At the age of 12, he started cross-referencing and catalog-

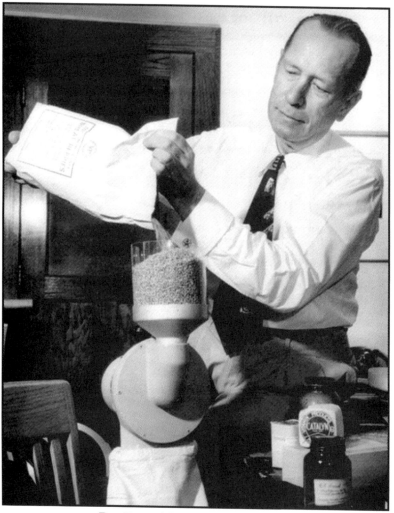

Dr. Royal Lee (1895 - 1967)

Perhaps the world's greatest nutritionist, Dr. Lee was also a prolific electronic inventor. Here he is working on his famous Lee Flour Mill. He designed it so the average household could have wholesome, fresh, low-heat, stone-ground flour with vitamin-rich germ and fiber-full bran intact. The Lee Foundation for Nutritional Research was a lighthouse as food adulteration and commercialism swept the twentieth century.

Photo and caption by permission of Mark Anderson

ing all nutritional references in this country, which he finished by his 16th birthday. For the next 50 years, Dr. Lee increased the scope of his knowledge to encyclopedic proportions on the subjects of health, nutrition, and medicine. He established The Lee Foundation for Nutritional Research which became one of the largest clearinghouses, worldwide, supporting practitioners in their quest for knowledge about health and nutrition. (After Dr. Lee's death, the vast educational material that he had published, along with copyrights for works by Drs. Wiley, Harrower, and Hawkins faded into obscurity. Today, the stewardship has been entrusted to the International Foundation for Nutrition and Health, www.ifnh.org)

In 1937, at the same time Dr. Lee was in court fighting the FDA to be able to advertise Zypan™ (the hydrochloric acid tablet he designed to help with digestion), Camel™ cigarettes was able to advertise in *Life* magazine that smoking cigarettes would promote digestion. This Camel ad can be seen in *Empty Harvest* and it shows a Thanksgiving meal divided into five courses, with short blurbs on how smoking in between each course will "help your digestion to run smoothly." [22]

A food editor, Miss Dorothy Malone, is pictured in one corner of the ad saying, "It's smart to have Camels on the table. My own personal experience is that smoking Camels with my meals and afterwards builds up a sense of digestive well-being." [23] The cigarette ad went on to say, "Enjoy Camels all you wish — all through the day." [24]

How many people were powerfully persuaded to smoke cigarettes because of advertising? Many people feel that if it is advertised, it is gospel. Advertising creates fads and trends. Today, cigarette companies would never be allowed to make such claims. Hundreds of thousands of people with lung cancer and emphysema followed this type of advertising advice.

What about another ad, from 1955, that claims that "Science shows how sugar can help keep your appetite — and weight

— under control." [25]

This ad actually promoted elevating blood sugar to cut down the sensation of hunger. Millions of people have become diabetics following such fallacious advice. These and many other misleading ads were allowed to be printed by the FDA.

From the early 1950s onward, Dr. Lee was constantly in federal court, trying to get the right to advertise his whole food nutritional products. If this sounds upside down, it is.

Dr. Lee and other pioneers, such as Drs. Weston Price, Melvin Page, and Francis Pottenger, tried to expose the rampant malnutrition in our nation, which was being caused by over-processed, dead, devitalized foods. They pointed out how tooth decay, diabetes, and arthritis, as well as other degenerative diseases, are *caused* by refined carbohydrates and sugars. Because Dr. Lee was so outspoken, he found himself branded as a racketeer and a quack ... just for promoting the therapeutic use of whole, natural, unadulterated foods with their vitamins and minerals intact.

Dr. Lee's goal was to give the public a way of somehow getting the vitamins and minerals that were removed from foods by over-processing. He believed that these factors were the reasons for the epidemic of coronary heart attacks that were sweeping the country in the early 1920s.

As Dr. Lee's and other voices were muzzled and gagged, the marketplace became filled with over-processed grains and cereals that in the mid-1940s had artificial vitamins added back into them, all for huge profits. "The newsletter of The Center for Science in the Public Interest, *Nutritional Action* (Vol. 16, No. 1), reports that the only difference between General Mills' *Wheaties™* and *Total™* cereals is that 1.5 cents' worth of synthetic vitamins are sprayed on *Total*. *Total* is then sold for 65 cents more than *Wheaties* This practice alone has generated $425 million in additional profits since 1972 for General Mills." [26]

Sadly, these huge profits mean that millions of people have ingested untold pounds of chemicalized and enriched food. Sadly

also, the world that Dr. Wiley, Dr. Lee, and others envisioned was not allowed to be.

A Word Or Two About Oils

"One hundred years ago, heart attacks were practically unheard of in the United States. The first recorded case of arteriosclerosis was in 1910; the first reported heart attack was in 1912. Alzheimer's disease did not exist. One person in 100,000 had diabetes. Now about two-thirds of Americans develop arteriosclerosis; 50% die of cardiovascular disease. One in 20 has some form of diabetes. One in four (28%) develops cancer – 500,000 of them die. Other degenerative conditions which have exploded in numbers since the turn of the century include multiple sclerosis, kidney degeneration, liver degeneration and others. One hundred years ago, people ate fresh, whole foods including plenty of meat, butter and lard. But they did not ordinarily eat any refined, processed or chemicalized foods, did not eat any refined and altered oils or fats. All of these are now commonly consumed." [27]

Many of the steps used to process vegetable oils can affect the nutritional content and balance of these products. Expeller-pressed oils and hydraulic-pressed oils are first subjected to temperatures of 200 degrees Fahrenheit and up. The oils are then de-gummed, which removes chlorophyll, vitamin E, lecithin and many minerals and trace elements. Then an alkaline wash separates out even more nutrients. Next, the oil is bleached and then deodorized by steam distillation at temperatures over 450 degrees F.

"The resulting oil is colorless, tasteless, odorless, altered and, of course, devoid of nutrients. Any vitamin complexes in the original food are gone; any possible remnants of nutrients are only fractions." [28]

Poisons Found In Refined Oils

The raw materials for oils now come from large, chemically-farmed fields. Very often, these over-refined oils contain pesticide residue, which interferes with nerve function and oxidation processes in the human body. These pesticide residues are only some of the toxic substances that are found in altered oils.

Trans-fatty acids, another toxic substance, make up, on the average, almost 10% of the total fats in the American diet. Trans-fatty acids are made by forcing hydrogen into raw, polyunsaturated oil molecules under high temperature and pressure. The oil is chemically altered so that the oil is more solid. This makes pastries flakier, breads moister, and cookies fresher-tasting. It also gives foods a longer shelf life.

Nutritional researcher, John Finnegan, states in his book *The Facts About Fats*: "There is more and more evidence showing that the main cause of heart disease and one of the main causes of cancer is the harmful effects from poisonous trans-fats and other compounds in refined oils."

The FDA recently announced that by January 1, 2006, nutrition labels will have to be changed to display the amount in grams of trans-fats that are included in each serving. We have to ask ourselves why the FDA is allowing these dangerous trans-fats in foods in the first place. To place them on a "nutrient" label shows just how lost the FDA really is. The new labels won't tell people how much of a trans-fats is too much. *Any* trans-fat is too much.

If you are confused about how to identify trans-fatty acids, here are the key markers:

1. The words "partially hydrogenated" are included in the list of ingredients on a product. Margarine, "composed of diacetyl, isopropyl, stearyl citrates, sodium benzoate, benzoic or citric acid, diglycerides and monoglycerides, is also loaded with

trans-fats. The Harvard School of Public Health found that just four servings of white bread, cake, or cookies that contain partially hydrogenated oils can increase the chance of heart trouble by 67%…2 ½ pats of margarine can increase it by 100%." [29]

2. Look for oil that is packaged in a clear bottle. Sunlight can penetrate and cause the oil to go rancid. Unfortunately, you will even find these in most health food stores where almost all "are usually manufactured by the same refineries as supermarket oils." [30] Buy oil in cans or dark brown glass bottles.

3. Smell your oils. Oils that are odorless and tasteless are rancid. Fresh, natural oils have their own delicate flavor and aroma.

We need the unsaturated fatty acids from good oils for many reasons: healthy skin and hair, maintenance of normal growth, hormone production, proper digestion, wound healing, calcium metabolism, etc. We have to be careful to choose good oils, like fresh flax seed oils and fish oils, to get the job done,.

Water — The Crucial Commodity

Both the endocrine system and the immune system are the most vitamin-and-mineral- dependent of all the systems in our bodies. One of the worst poisons our glands can encounter, *sodium fluoride,* was added to most municipal drinking for decades. Calcium fluoride, a naturally-occurring form of fluoride found in well water in trace amounts, *was not* the form of fluoridation chosen by the municipalities. Sodium fluoride is a highly toxic by-product of aluminum production and can destroy the enzymes that make vitamins work in your body.

As if sodium fluoride wasn't toxic enough, the substance that is now used in 90% of the water fluoridation programs today is

fluosilicic acid, which is actually classified as a hazardous waste. Fluosilicic acid is derived from the "pollution scrubbing devices of the super phosphate fertilizer industry, 70 to 75% of which comes from the Cargill fertilizer corporation. The only other place this fluosilicic acid can be disposed of is a hazardous waste facility." [31] At this facility, it would have to be neutralized at a cost of $1.40 per gallon or more.

We have to be aware that we are allowing industries to sell their toxic waste to our municipal water districts. These industries are actually making money on toxic waste that they don't want to pay to have neutralized and disposed.

In 1997, the union representing all toxicologists, chemists, biologists, and other professionals at the Environmental Protection Agency voted to support a California initiative to stop fluoridation of public drinking water. The reason was the growing evidence that the type of fluoridation used, *fluosilicic acid*, actually causes:

1. Depression of the thyroid. Thyroid disease is the most common glandular disorder, affecting approximately 20 million Americans. "Insufficient thyroid hormones causes all bodily functions to slow down…the symptoms of hypothyroidism are subtle and gradual and may be mistaken for depression."[32] These symptoms can manifest as weight gain, headaches, poor memory and concentration, hair loss, etc. The thyroid also helps the body to adapt between heat and cold. When it is unresponsive, people's bodies cannot respond appropriately to the temperature changes that winter or summer bring. This results in unprocessed metabolic waste accumulating in their systems. This toxic waste strains the immune system, and the person gets a cold or the flu.

2. Hip fractures for both older men and women. A study published in the Journal of the American Medical Association in 1990 concluded that drinking fluoridated water will double

the number of hip fractures for this group.

3. Hormone disruption. FDA scientists reported in the Journal of Toxicology and Environmental Health in 1994 that there was a close correlation between decreasing total fertility rates in women between the ages of 10 and 49, and increasing fluoride levels. (Interestingly, fluosilicic acid as fluoride is an unapproved new drug as far as the FDA is concerned. The FDA also does not consider fluoride an essential nutrient, yet it is allowed to be added to our drinking water.)

It is important to remember that drinking a good quality water is important to your health in many ways.

2/Synthetic Vitamins vs. Food

"I had a letter from an Austrian colleague who was suffering from a severe hemorrhagic diathesis (infection). He wanted to try ascorbic acid in (for) his condition. Possessing at that time no sufficient quantities of crystalline ascorbic acid, I sent him a preparation of paprika that contained much ascorbic acid and the man was cured by it. Later, with my friend, St. Rusznyak, we tried to produce the same therapeutical effect in similar conditions with pure ascorbic acid, but we obtained no response. It was evident that the action of paprika was due to some other substance present in this plant."

— *Albert von Szent-Gyorgi*
Hungarian-born U.S. biochemist; Nobel Prize winner
for discovering that vitamin C cured scurvy

The FDA has claimed for years that foods are not therapeutic. *Funk & Wagnall's* definition of *therapeutic* is: "Having healing qualities; curative." The early nutritional pioneers believed that whole foods were the *only* foundation for optimum health, and, as such, were also the main foundation for a return to health. I agree with them. However, the dismissal of the therapeutic value of whole foods made it possible for the FDA and our lawmakers to support a commercial food industry staggering in its size and revenues. As a result, this has left you and me with a health crisis that is out of control.

In an attempt to help themselves, most people run to their local drugstore or health food store and grab some synthetic vitamins off the shelf. Others may call on a friend or go on the web to get

the latest cure in a multi-level marketing scheme. If one listens carefully to multi-level marketing information on nutrition, they often claim to have now isolated THE nutrient factor that will save mankind. But what they don't know is that, in the long run, they may be compounding their health problems and their customers' by taking synthetic versions of vitamins.

The truth is, when you purchase synthetic vitamins, you are really only getting more of what is already being dumped into our food supply under the guise of enrichment. "Enrich" is defined by *Webster's Dictionary* as, "To improve the quality of: to make a valuable addition to." But, let's take a look at some of these synthetic vitamins and see if they really improve the quality of a food.

When you look at a loaf of enriched bread, it will say "enriched flour (barley malt, ferrous sulfate (iron), "B" vitamins (niacin, thiamine mononitrate, (B_1), riboflavin (B_2), folic acid)." *The Consumer's Dictionary of Food Additives* by Ruth Winter, M.S., states that *ferrous sulfate* is used as "a wood preservative, weed killer, and to treat anemia." Thiamine mononitrate comes from coal tar. If you heated a B vitamin made from this substance with a blowtorch, it would turn into a glob of tar, much like the tar on your roof.

How can refined and processed coal tar be called a vitamin, when, in fact, vitamins were discovered in live foods? How can such a source be called "natural" or "organic?" Let's take a look at the FDA definitions for these terms:

- Natural — Anything that ultimately comes from nature, including chemicals, since they ultimately come from nature (coal tar is *natural*).
- Organic — Anything that contains a carbon molecule (DDT has a carbon base and could be labeled *organic*).

By leaving these terms ambiguous, it leaves room for abuse

by the unscrupulous. Is this what we had in mind when we purchased a "natural" vitamin, or an "organic" supplement? Or did we imagine a farm where no pesticides are used and the land is fertilized with composting? Well, that is not the way it is.

Why Natural Food Complexes Faded From View

In the beginning of vitamin research, almost all of the scientific experiments used natural, food-sourced nutrients, and a lot was learned. In fact, almost all the studies done showing that vitamins really work were done with food-source nutrients. In studies that show that vitamins don't work, a synthetic is *always* used. Nutrients are difficult for the FDA and other agencies to control. But isolating vitamins and standardizing them as drugs gives them a means of controlling them.

"For the pharmaceutical companies, vitamin fractions such as vitamin A, vitamin C, beta-carotene, and vitamin E; trace minerals such as zinc and selenium (usually sold in inorganic and imbalanced forms), coenzyme Q, and many other specific nutrients can be cheaply manufactured and sold at huge profits." [33]

In her book, *The Real Truth About Vitamins and Antioxidants,* Judith DeCava, a noted nutritional author, talks about the "standard medical view," which is an "attempt to blend medicine with nutrition, using chemically-isolated nutrients as drugs." Ms. DeCava makes some important points:

1. "Medical schools in this country are now standardized (if not homogenized) and no matter what medical school one attends, one gets essentially the same instruction …" [34]
2. "Doctors believe that their education gives them a strange sort of infallibility to lend their expertise in areas of medicine for which they have received no training, as in nutrition, leading them to discount ideas and even valid research." [35] This is supported by the fact that in 1991, only 22 out of the 127

accredited U. S. medical schools required a single course in nutrition.

3. From World War II onward, nutritional information was based on research studies funded by the special interests of the different pharmaceutical companies, which manufactured fractionated, crystalline-pure, and synthetic chemicals. This biased information became pretty much all that appeared in medical journals, newspapers, TV, and radio. The average person has no idea what the real sources of synthetic vitamins are, which has led to a lot of absurdity, because people take these in the belief that they are making up for what is lost in their food. So, unfortunately, the average person today accepts that a vitamin made from coal tar is healthy and beneficial for him. (For more information about how these synthetic vitamins are made, visit my website, www.theperfectcrime.com.)

Cellular malnutrition as a cause of disease has been avoided in orthodox medicine, while synthetic vitamins, which have drug-like effects, have been embraced. Often, these synthetics actually contaminate the internal environment of the body. But these synthetics, unlike whole food concentrates, can be easily mass-produced by large pharmaceutical companies, who can store and distribute them. As a result, these isolated synthetics are used in nearly all nutritional supplements, whether found in a drug store, health food store, or nutritionist's office.

Just What Are Natural Complexes?

Vitamins are "groups of chemically related compounds." There is a part that is identified as the organic nutrient of the vitamin, i.e., ascorbic acid *as* vitamin C. But then there are enzymes, co-enzymes, antioxidants, trace elements, activators, and other unknown factors that enable the vitamin to go into biochemical operation (See diagrams on the next page). In other words,

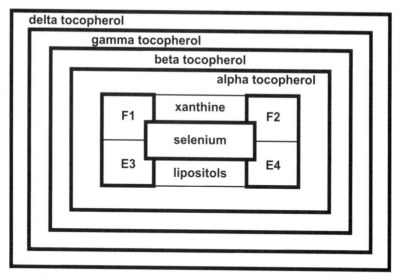

The Functional Architecture of the Vitamin E Complex

Reprinted with permission from Judith DeCava

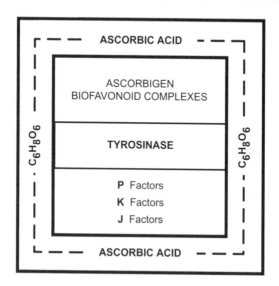

**The Functional Architecture
of Vitamin C Complex**

Reprinted with permission from Judith DeCava

33

ascorbic acid is a *part* of the vitamin C complex. It is *not*, all by itself, vitamin C.

"With foods and food concentrates — containing whole nutritional complexes — the body can choose its needs for assimilation and excrete what it does not need; this is called 'selective absorption.' On the other hand, with fractionated or isolated and/or synthetic vitamins, there is no choice; the body must handle the chemical in some manner and can suffer consequences of biochemical imbalances and toxic overdose." [36]

The living vitamin complex of foods cannot be taken apart and re-assembled and be expected to work the way it did before. In fact, it won't work at all; yet, this is exactly what has been done to produce crystalline-pure, fractionated vitamins.

Once the vitamin complex has been separated into its components and is dead and inert, it is then that the "scientific method" takes it and develops trials or experiments.

"Synthetic, fractionated, crystalline-pure vitamins are not whole, natural compounds; they are not food which human systems can utilize as nutrients, with which human systems are familiar, and which will not disrupt normal biochemistry. How could any scientist say that the body does not know the difference between natural and synthetic vitamins?" [37] (Especially now that you know what synthetic vitamins are actually made from.)

What has happened is "true science is now judged on the basis of an experimental method which measures, classifies, and duplicates reactions and effects of single chemicals. This rules out testing natural vitamin complexes … This also rules out clinical observation — seeing how a patient is doing and communicating with him/her as to individual benefits, needs and responses." [38]

People do not understand that the rules and parameters used in testing vitamins from the 1960s on pretty much eliminates the use of any natural food-based product in these tests. Once again, you can't patent wheat germ oil or liver or yeast and make huge profits. But you can patent micro-parts of oils and coal tar and

make enormous profits.

The government has supported this narrow view for decades. "Indeed, FDA officials have consistently tended to leave out of their thinking both the human element in disease and the idea that cellular malnutrition is a prominent cause of disease." [39]

Rats And The RDAs (Recommended Daily Allowances)

The "scientific studies" I have previously mentioned substitute synthetic, crystalline-pure vitamins for whole food complexes, and ignore the human element by substituting rats, chicks and rabbits for humans. A zoo would *never* feed all the different animals the same food or the same proportions, yet the RDA for humans is now based on Rat Bioassay.

"The bioassay method is based upon the direct measurement of a vitamin's biological activity in preventing or curing certain specific pathological (disease) conditions in a predetermined experimental animal ... This method expresses measurement, in terms of units. So, the amount found to alleviate disease in the rat or other laboratory animal is "translated" into the amount and form needed for humans." [40]

Rats are scavengers. Humans are not. The very physiological makeup of lower animals enables them to eat, digest and utilize foods and rubbish which we cannot. And here is the kicker:

"... Laboratory animals fed ascorbic acid — the manufactured, chemically-pure fraction of the vitamin C complex — can convert that chemical into the required vitamin C complex. Such animals with scurvy, when fed ascorbic acid, may improve so that symptoms are relieved. Humans with scurvy, when fed ascorbic acid, do not improve very much, if at all." [41] In fact, if we look at Szent-Gyorgi's quote at the beginning of this chapter, we realize that ascorbic acid couldn't cure his colleague from severe bleeding, but paprika did.

Getting To The Core Of The Matter

Now we come to the reason why synthetic or crystalline-pure vitamins are *not* good for you. Guess what? They're not real. But, here is why they could actually harm you. Take, for example, ascorbic acid as vitamin C. If a person has sufficient reserves of the other components of the C complex (enzymes, co-enzymes, antioxidants, trace element activators and other unknown factors), to recombine and process an intake of ascorbic acid, that person will experience some improvement for a time. When these reserves are drained, the ascorbic acid will no longer benefit that person. The very symptoms that the person was trying to eliminate will return, and the person will then have a full-blown vitamin C deficiency.

The body treats all synthetic vitamins as foreign substances, reacting to them like toxins. These toxins are then processed and neutralized by the liver, which sends them to the kidneys for elimination. This is the real story behind the "expensive urine" of excessive vitamin intake that we hear so much about.

Many people feel an energy increase, often euphoria, when they start to take synthetic vitamins. But, taking excessive amounts for an extended period will cause the effects to reverse. Take, for example, synthetic Thiamine (B_1). It "will initially allay fatigue but will eventually *cause* fatigue by the build-up of pyruvic acid. This leads to the vicious cycle of thinking more and more Thiamine is needed, resulting in more and more fatigue along with other accumulated complaints." [42]

Because of the different amounts of stored reserves people have, there are two situations that sincere nutritionists in whole complex research keep pointing out:

1. Vitamins cannot be standardized, because there is no way to determine what different people's needs are, and there is no way to calculate their reserves.

2. An individual's ability to process, recombine and eliminate synthetic vitamins are full of contradictory effects (i.e., good, bad or indifferent effects).

Whole, Natural Vitamins vs. Synthetic

Judith DeCava said it succinctly: "Regardless of the seemingly good initial response, using 'high potency' synthetic vitamins will, in time, bring a person into that 'intermediate zone' where the effects begin to reverse. This partially explains the confusion between natural and synthetic vitamins." [43] Ms. DeCava goes into different studies comparing whole, natural vs. synthetic vitamins. The whole, natural ones always come up ahead. But, do we, as consumers, know what is natural and what is not? If the labeling of "natural" is so subjective and undefined, how can one tell the difference?

The named source of the vitamin is the best clue. So, for your information, the following is a list of the most common synthetic forms of vitamins. You might want to take this book and make a copy of the following chart in order to compare this list to the vitamins and foods you have in your kitchen cupboards. (Check your pet foods, too!) Keep in mind that synthetic vitamins, which are legally considered to be the same in nutritional value and cheaper to make, are the ones mainly used.

We are also used to seeing listings in high milligram potency; however, we need to remember that a high number of milligrams is also an indication of a synthetic source.

The B vitamins should be taken as a whole, with all members of the group. In nature, all the Bs are always found together — never is one isolated from the rest.

Dr. Royal Lee said in his *Vitamin News* that "a natural combination of vitamin B complex, a complete source in natural balance including intact synergists, is from 10 to 50 times more *potent* in humans, unit for unit, than is a chemically purified or

VITAMIN	SYNTHETIC VITAMIN	FOOD-BASED VITAMINS
Vitamin A	Acetate Retinal Palmitate Beta Carotene	Fish oils Liver Carrot powder
Vitamin B_1	Thiamine HCl Thiamine Mononitrate	Nutritional yeast
Vitamin B_3	Niacin	Nutritional yeast, liver
Vitamin C	Ascorbic Acid Pycnogenols	Green leafy vegetables Buckwheat juice, citrus
Vitamin D	Irradiated Ergosterol	Cholecalciferol, fish oil
Vitamin E	d-Alpha Tocopherol dl-Alpha Tocopherol d-Alpha Succinate	Wheat germ oil Green leafy vegetables Peavine plant

synthetic complex… No ONE source contains ALL the factors of the complete B complex, and for highest potency a number of therapeutically active sources must be tapped." [44]

Dr. Lee listed 22 factors and synergists present in his B complex. By tapping so many different food sources, he was able to include vitamin B_4, which he called the anti-paralysis factor. He said that a deficiency in vitamin E can result in muscle tissue degeneration of the heart, and a deficiency of vitamin B_4 can result in a heart block, due to the degeneration of the nerves in the heart muscle. BOTH the B and E complexes were always consumed by people when cereal grains were whole and contained the cereal germ.

Dr. Lee noted that the 22 different factors and synergists in his Cataplex B combined into 50 to 100 isomers. The molecular complexity of this is mind-boggling, and he stressed the fact that

to attempt to synthesize or tamper chemically with *extremely complicated* food factors is futile. I say it's ridiculous.

Standard Process lists on its Cataplex B (Cataplex means whole food complex) the following milligrams per three tablets:

Thiamine:	0.95 mg
Niacin:	20.44 mg
Vitamin B_6:	0.95 mg

This is a far cry from the majority of B complexes on the market, which range from 50 – 100 mg for each synthesized B, with all of the complexity of food factors missing.

Cataplex B does not list every B however, because the rest of the B complex is present in small, potent, food-based amounts that the FDA has no approved labeling for. The FDA only recognizes milligrams based on synthetic vitamins.

Potency Is Not Milligrams Or Micrograms Or Units

Potency is defined as "the strength, ability, or capacity to bring about a particular result." [45] Unfortunately, to the general public, potency is taken to mean high milligrams or units of synthetic vitamins. These "high potency" vitamins require a large amount of the fractured vitamin to achieve a specific reaction; although, as previously mentioned, not necessarily a nutritional reaction. In fact, *a minute amount of a vitamin in its whole food form is more effective nutritionally than a large amount of a synthetic one.*

Let us take a look at a story about a medical doctor held captive in a North Korean prisoner of war camp during the Korean War (1950-1953). After a period of time with an inadequate diet, many of the doctor's fellow prisoners of war began to show signs of beriberi, a disease that results from a severe thiamine (B_1) deficiency. He notified the Red Cross, and they sent him some vitamin B_1, in the synthetic form, Thiamine HCL. The doctor gave

this to his patients, but their health continued to deteriorate. This puzzled him, since B_1 was the medical treatment recommended in the *Materia Medica*.

The doctor's North Korean guards whispered to him that the beriberi could be cured by using rice polish, the nutritive-rich germ of the rice that is removed when rice is refined. He thought it was absurd, but he had nothing to lose, so he started giving his patients a teaspoon or more of rice polish every day. Within a short time, his patients' symptoms started to abate and the beriberi plague ceased.

It is important to note that it would take a ton (2,000 pounds) of unmilled rice to produce a level teaspoon of thiamine (B_1)! The amount the prisoners of war were getting would equate to the amount on the head of a pin. This is a great example of how potent whole foods are. It is also an excellent example of how nutritious a food like rice can be in its whole form; yet, most people eat white rice with nearly all the vitamins removed.

Synthetics Are Not As Effective

Vitamin E "loses up to 99% of its potency when separated from its natural synergists." [46] When you take just the tocopherols, you are throwing out the real vitamin E. The tocopherols are nature's way of protecting and preserving vitamin E, similar to the way the peel of a banana protects the contents.

"In one test study, the vitamin E-deficient laboratory animals fed tocopherols died sooner than the control animals that received no vitamins at all." [47]

In another study, "Silver foxes were fed a synthetic diet so that every component of the diet would be known. The animals were given all of the known B vitamins — in synthetic form — but they did not grow; their fur deteriorated, and finally they died. Another group of foxes on the same diet were given a change after a short time: added to their rations were yeast and liver, both sources of

natural whole B complex. These animals grew normally and the quality of their fur improved with their health." [48]

Many people reach for ascorbic acid when they have a cold. Yet, "modern-day studies, utilizing ascorbic acid (the crystalline-pure fraction) rather than vitamin C complex, find the synthetic fraction has virtually *no* effect on pneumonia, bronchitis, or other pulmonary problems even though sufferers show low serum levels of vitamin C ... daily intake of ascorbic acid supplements reduces the total white blood cell count, compromising the immune response rather than assisting it." [49]

Confusion about ascorbic acid is created by reports of how it has helped to fight colds and infections in *short-term* use. Dr. Bernard Jensen points out in *Empty Harvest* that "the answer probably lies more in ascorbic acid's pH balance influence (acid/alkaline balance) than any other factor." [50]

Since most infectious bacteria thrive in an alkaline pH, high consumption of ascorbic acid when first catching a cold then creates an acid environment in which the bacteria cannot thrive. Dr. D. C. Jarvis, in his book, *Folk Medicine*, talks about the importance of the acid/alkaline balance in the body's immune system. Jarvis promotes the intake of 2-3 tablespoons of apple cider vinegar daily. New studies have shown that apple cider vinegar can help people to lose weight by stimulating the parasympathetic nervous system. It also helps to promote calcium and magnesium absorption and stimulates pancreatic function. Apple cider vinegar is 5% *acetic acid*, which is normally found in the body.

Over and over again, it has been proven that the natural, whole food complexes that Mother Nature created are perfectly balanced to work with human physiology to correct a vast number of disorders. However, it is to be emphasized here that a good diet is the basis of health, and supplements are the means of catching up for lost time nutritionally.

Antioxidants — The Controversy

The controversy over the need for antioxidants has been going on for some time. Those who advocate the need for antioxidants usually know nothing about whole food complexes. Remember, most of the news on vitamins from 1962 onward has been "nearly or entirely all based on studies using the fractionated, crystalline-pure, synthetic chemicals." [51]

Antioxidants are the part of the vitamin complex that prevent or inhibit oxidation. Vitamin E is a natural part of polyunsaturated fatty acids and protects oils from deteriorating. In fact, if the oil is rancid, it indicates that the vitamins E, A, and carotenes have been destroyed. And, vitamin E (d-alpha tocopherols), vitamin C (ascorbic acid), and beta-carotene are the most widely touted antioxidants.

"Using antioxidants alone as nutritional supplements means ingesting fractions, isolated substances, not whole complexes. It would be like eating the peel of a banana without the banana, or like eating the shell of a nut without the nut meat." [52]

To make matters worse, most commercial antioxidants are produced in pharmaceutical manufacturing plants. "Hoffman-LaRouche, for example, a huge pharmaceutical (drug) conglomerate, is building a plant in Freeport, Texas, to turn out 350 tons of synthetic Beta-carotene, enough to supply a six milligram capsule daily to every American adult every year." [53] No, there are not truckloads of carrots or any other natural food source going to that plant. Except, of course, possibly in the workers' lunchboxes.

This crystalline-pure form of beta-carotene cannot perform as a nutrient. To attribute the beneficial effects of fruits and vegetables to a single food component, such as carotenes, is useless. There are 50 to 60 carotenes found in the typical American diet, and "humans need complex food sources of even similar or related nutrients, this according to individual needs at specific times." [54]

We hear much talk about "free radicals" attacking human

cells and weakening our immune systems. Oxidation is a process whereby a molecule contains one or more unpaired electrons (Atoms contain a nucleus, protons, neutrons and electrons. The electrons move around the nucleus in pairs.). In the free radical theory, these molecules try to pick up an electron from another molecule, thus starting a chain reaction.

However, as Judith DeCava's studies point out, most honest scientists know that "every compound excreted by the body is in one form or another bound to oxygen for elimination." [55]

In simple terms, oxidation is nature's way of eliminating cellular waste and debris. It is also nature's way of dealing with tissues that are injured by removing damaged cells. So, why are we making such a deal about preventing this when it's a necessary process?

Antioxidants As A Fad

Most of the scientific research on synthesized antioxidants has been performed in test tubes or on microscopic slides. What is overlooked is the human body's ability to absorb them. (Just a small issue!) With the emphasis on profit, a vast majority of studies are not performed on humans. So how can anyone promote unknown benefits?

In fact, too many synthetic antioxidants can cause fatigue and muscle weakness. Denham Harman, M.D., PhD., the "father" of the free radical theory of aging, was asked about the antioxidant vitamins he takes. "Dr. Harman listed an amazingly small amount compared to what many in the nutrition field are recommending: a maximum of 400 IU of 'vitamin E' (alpha-tocopherol) daily, 2,000 mg of 'vitamin C' (ascorbic acid) daily, and 25,000 IU of beta-carotene every other day. 'I'd take more', he said, 'but I can't afford to be fatigued.'" [56]

Toxic effects from large intakes of synthetic antioxidants have been reported, a scary effect from supplements that are supposed

to prevent disease and aging. Natural food complexes do not cause adverse effects.

Antioxidants are widely promoted for all of us to take, yet:

1. The process, oxidation, that synthetic antioxidants are supposed to protect us from, is a *natural by-product of cellular combustion*. Without it, we would be dead.
2. When taken in large doses, synthetic antioxidants cause fatigue and muscular weakness.
3. When taken in even larger doses, these synthetic antioxidants are toxic.

This is a prime example of a "new medical fact" that has become an accepted way of thinking for nutritionally-minded people. If this is not a fad, what is?

Fads, Trends And Bold-Faced Lies

Fad is defined by *Webster's Dictionary* as, "an exaggeratedly fussy attitude, especially about eating or not eating certain kinds of food." My definition of a "fad" is:

1. You keep eating a certain way, even though you look and feel worse.
2. You keep eating a certain way, because it is advertised and talked about, even though you look and feel worse.
3. You know all of the "scientific reasons" for eating this way, even though you look and feel worse.

All of these definitions certainly fit into our times today. People keep taking synthetic vitamins and wondering why there is no noticeable improvement in their health over the long haul, and why they don't feel as good as they used to.

Webster defines a *trend* as, "a dominant movement revealed

by a statistical process." Americans have been on an unnatural trend in their food sources for nearly 100 years.

"As a culture, we are not just unnatural — it is deeper. We are anti-natural." [57] But most people do not understand that this is what we have become as a result of catchy slogans and slick marketing that cover up the dangers created by Wall Street greed.

Bold-faced is defined by Webster as, "showing an impudent lack of shame." An impudent lack of shame is evident by those who proclaim that the human body cannot tell the difference between natural and synthetic vitamins and foods.

Why Do I Need Vitamins And Minerals If I'm Eating Well?

Vitamins are factors that cause health.

Vitamins act as facilitators in all of the chemical reactions in the body. Because most people have likes and dislikes that keep them from eating green, leafy vegetables such as kale, broccoli, and other foods necessary for good health, vitamin supplements are a must.

Because of the commercial food industry and its farming and processing techniques, which remove most of the nutrients from foods, Americans found themselves early on consuming a very poor diet. By the 1930s, the food supply had become predominantly bleached, refined, chemically preserved, pasteurized, sterilized, and homogenized. The nutritional deficiencies which these foods created caused "… the previously unanticipated phenomenon of many genetically transmitted conditions, because they originated in deficiency and poisoning patters of forbearers." [58]

Dr. Royal Lee said in 1950, "Trace mineral deficiency, it is evident, can act also to impair hereditary transmission. As these trace minerals and determinants (cell blueprints) are combined organically into protein linkages, it is evident how the nature of these minerals in our foods is of vital importance. Compost

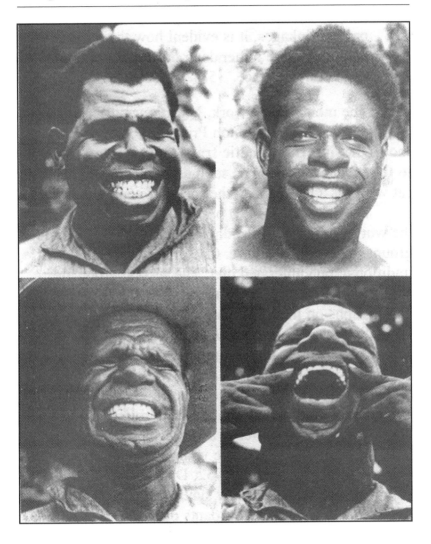

Natives on the islands of the Great Barrier Reef. The dental arches here reach a high degree of excellence.

Photos and captions by permission of the Price-Pottenger Foundation, California

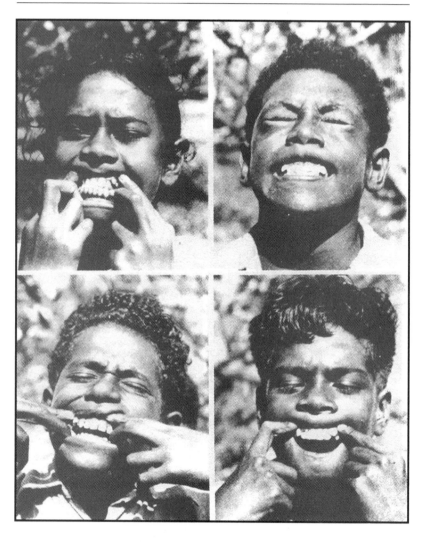

The contrast between the primitive and modernized natives in facial and dental arch form is as striking here as elsewhere. These young natives were born to parents who had adopted our modern foods of commerce. Note the narrowed faces and dental arches with pinched nostrils and crowding of the teeth. Their magnificent heredity could not protect them.

Photos and captions by permission of the Price-Pottenger Foundation, California

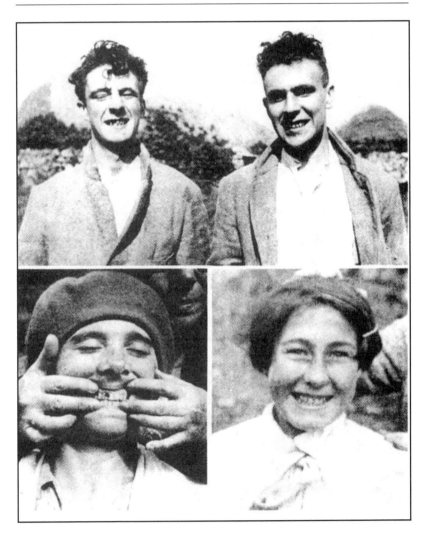

Above: brothers, Isle of Harris. The younger at left uses modern food and has rampant tooth decay. Brother at right uses native food and has excellent teeth. Not narrowed face and arch of younger brother. Below left: typical rampant tooth decay, modernized Gaelic. Below right: typical excellent teeth of primitive Gaelic.

Photos and captions by permission of the Price-Pottenger Foundation, California

gardening [organic gardening] in building up the organic mineral levels of the soil is here justified." [59]

The monumental work, *Nutrition and Physical Degeneration*, by Weston Price, D.D.S., graphically shows that inferior genetic traits were passed along to the next generation as soon as the parents began to eat what Dr. Price called "the foods of commerce."

Dr. Price traveled to primitive cultures around the world in the 1930s and photographed two different groups within each culture. One group ate its traditional, unadulterated diet. The second group ate civilized counterfeit and adulterated foods.

Dr. Price estimated that the group who ate an unadulterated diet consumed at least 4 to 10 times more of the amounts of vitamins and minerals everyday than did the group who ate processed and refined foods. That is between 1,500 and 3,650 lost nutrients in one year. Over a period of 10 years, the loss is HUGE. (How can this *not* affect our health?) Dr. Price found that this loss of vitamins and minerals kept various organs from being nourished and prevented perfect heredity from happening by altering the genes. No wonder whole food supplements are so important for us today.

So, basically we are the second, third and fourth generations in this over-processed and ruined diet transmission. We are in need of as much nutritional building as we can possibly get. To continue to consume synthetic vitamins to build up an immune system already weakened by depleted foods and synthetic vitamins will not work. (The equation of more of nothing does not equal more of anything.)

In fact, these synthetic vitamins are often poisonous. In January of 1952, Dr. Lee announced: "I could write volumes on how synthetic vitamins, like thiamine, castrate the descendants of the victim who uses even as much as double the daily requirement." [60]

Dr. Lee then cited a study by Dr. Barnett Sure (*Jol. Natr.*, August 1939). Dr. Sure studied "two groups of pigs, feeding

one group twice the daily requirements of synthetic B, and the other group the same amount of natural B. The result: *All* of the first generation offspring from the pigs fed the synthetic vitamin were *sterile*…obviously, synthetic B is NOT A NUTRIENT, it is a genetic poison that damages the chromosome packages responsible for transmitting sexual characteristics from the parent to the offspring." [61]

Humans, unlike pigs, take more than one generation to reap this genetic damage. A 1981 report from the University of Florida stated that the American male sperm count in 1929 was at approximately 100 million sperm cells per millimeter of semen. By 1973 the sperm count had dropped to 60 million per millimeter. Then, seven years later, in 1980, the average count had dropped to 20 million per millimeter.

"What in the world happened to bring about such a horrible drop in male fertility in just 61 years? One very possible explanation could very well lie in the historical use of synthetic B and other counterfeit nutrients … Since World War II, the American people, and people of other countries as well, have had a daily ration of a genetic poison in most of the bread, flour products, cereals and other food items that are forced, by law, to enrich with the only cost-feasible enricher: *synthetic vitamins*." [62] (A dead food + a dead vitamin = a longer shelf life = more profits.)

A Word About Standard Process

Standard Process was an outgrowth of Dr. Royal Lee's passion for nutrition. In 1929, Dr. Lee's mother came down with a strange flu and was diagnosed with a bad heart. She was given six months to live. When Dr. Lee learned of this prognosis, he immediately went to work on a potent, concentrated multiple vitamin, trace mineral, and enzyme product. He brought his mother this potent vitamin and, very quickly, she began to improve. His mother lived for another 12 years (to her 80th birthday). Dr. Lee

soon named this vitamin Catalyn™, and it became the first product in the Standard Process line.

Every time a new trace mineral, enzyme, or micronutrient is discovered, it is discovered in foods. And, every time these discoveries are made, Catalyn is analyzed, and the newly discovered trace mineral, enzyme, or micronutrient is found to be in it. Why? Because Catalyn contains every possible whole food source that would support a person's biochemistry. And, as mentioned earlier, foods are not just composed of one thing — foods are a blend of *untold* numbers, types, and variations of nutrient complexes. Dr. Lee once said that it took him longer to develop a nutritional formula than to come up with one of his inventions because of the complexity of factors already present in nature.

As doctors would encounter some illness or disease in the field, Dr. Lee would go to his laboratory and develop a *whole food supplement* that would support a natural healing process. Thus, as an outpouring of Dr. Lee's great love of humanity, the entire Standard Process line came into being.

Because Dr. Lee insisted that foods were therapeutic, he was always in court fighting the FDA, which insisted that only drugs could be called therapeutic. (At one time, Standard Process was called the Therapeutic Food Company.) Finally, he was forced to allow all of his research to be destroyed. This included every copy of his *Therapeutic Food Manual, Product Bulletin*, *Vitamin News*, and numerous articles written for publication. He was also no longer allowed to speak on health, nutrition, or medicine, or he would go to jail for seven years. Consequently, all of the materials were burned. It's hard to believe that this happened in the United States in the early 1960s — instead of in Nazi Germany in 1939.

Remember what the German chemical industrialists did to Julius Hensel's book on rock dust? Hensel's book could not be found for many years and was squelched so that the consumers were lead to conclude that it was false. Fortunately for us, copies

of most of Dr. Lee's materials were stored in the archives of a non-profit organization and are now available from the International Foundation for Nutrition and Health.

Standard Process whole food supplements are made according to the rigid guidelines set by Dr. Lee. All of the natural foods used are grown on rich farmland that Dr. Lee chose specifically for its abundance of minerals left by a retreating glacier. He also chose the location in Wisconsin because of an aquifer of unlimited mineral-rich water underneath it. This thick, black topsoil has always been free from chemical fertilizers and pesticides. Dr. Lee's formulas are made from whole foods concentrated to clinical potency. For example, Standard Process takes 3,000 gallons of beets and concentrates them into a powder that could fit into a briefcase. This is then added to Standard Process' Betafood™ and AF Betafood™, which help the gall bladder function.

With Standard Process' Cataplex E™ (Cataplex means whole food complex), you get the E complex in the form that Dr. Lee discovered was the richest source of the E complex: the juice of the whole pea plant.

If this sounds weak or impotent, remember what potency really is: *The strength, ability, or capacity to bring about a particular result.*

These potent nutrients can help us to catch up for lost time nutritionally. What this catching up for lost time nutritionally really means is best illustrated by the following quote from Dr. Bruce West, whose well-known newsletter, *Health Alert*, has helped thousands of people on the road to health.

"If you had a heart problem with high blood fats and poor digestion, my best R_x would be some powerful dietary changes. For starters, if this was feasible, I would like to see you consume daily: a pound of raw, organic liver; a couple of buckets of organic wheat germ and high-selenium yeast; a small wheelbarrow full of organic beets and beet tops; gallons of freshly-squeezed vegetable juices; and plenty of raw, fresh-pressed organic oils,

such as flax seed oil. Naturally, this is impossible. So, instead we use supplements which are *condensed from these foods and other nutrients.*" [63]

Since Dr. Royal Lee believed that we, as humans, need the nutrition from both plants and animals, many Standard Process products have both. An example of this would be folic acid and vitamin B_{12}. Folic acid is derived from plants; vitamin B_{12} from liver. So Standard Process has carrot powder and bovine liver as their listed sources for these vitamins. All Standard Process products are tested and retested countless times by certified laboratory technicians to ensure the purity of all nutrients used.

The Work In Nutrition Has Already Been Done

Everything we need to know about nutrition has already been done by Mother Nature herself. Nature is the chemist, and all that a biochemist can do is to unlock the *already existing relationships* within and among all of these micronutrient factors, split them up, identify them, and test them to see what happens if a laboratory animal goes without them.

This happens on a regular basis. Every day a "new" discovery hits the news media. (Co-Enzyme Q-10, Co-enzyme PQQ, antioxidants, Selenium, Pycnogenols, Phyto-Chemicals, etc.)

The interesting fact is that Standard Process contains all of these "new" discoveries, because whole food supplements contain all of the synergists (enzymes, co-enzymes, trace minerals and all of the *unknown* factors yet to be discovered). By taking foods intact, you always get everything you need. You also do not have to play the guessing game of figuring out how much of a new discovery you need to take.

When you have a bottle of vitamin E (d-Alpha tocopherol), a bottle of Selenium, and a bottle of Co-enzyme Q-10, what you actually have are parts of the E complex that are being purchased separately. What you are actually getting is dead and inert. It is

impossible to get the dosages correct, and there are many other components which you are not getting.

A Sobering Word

J. I. Rodale, the American naturalist, wrote wisely in his classic work, *The Complete Book of Food and Nutrition*:

"We *must* take vitamins if we wish to be healthy and the nation as a whole must do it, or God alone knows what will happen to the second or third generations coming up — generations inheriting weaknesses passed on to them by us, generations which few of us will live to see unless we augment our diet with vitamins and minerals. And, as parting advice, don't take coal tar (synthetic) vitamins. Examine every bottle. Be sure that the vitamins you take are extracted from food. Scientific research proves that this is best." [64]

It couldn't have been said any better. Remember Thiamine HCL and Thiamine Mononitrate come from coal tar *and are in all commercial breads.* Vitamin B_{12} comes from activated sewage sludge and vitamin D is concocted from irradiated oil.

Bon Apetit.

3/Fats, Proteins, and Your Health

"If the members of the American Medical establishment were to have a collective find-yourself-standing-naked-in-Times-Square-nightmare, this might be it. They spend 30 years ridiculing Robert Atkins…accusing the Manhattan doctor of quackery and fraud, only to discover that the unrepentant Atkins was right all along. Or maybe it's this: They find that their very own dietary recommendations — eat less fat and more carbohydrates — are the cause of the rampaging epidemic of obesity in America. Or, just possibly this: They find out both of the above are true."

Gary Taubes
"What If It's Been A Big Fat Lie"
New York Times Magazine, July 7, 2002

With our food supply polluted and our synthetic vitamins in hand, what else can be done to ruin our health? Well, we could be encouraged to eat a diet low in fats and protein and high in carbohydrates, thus ensuring that we ingest *more refined, chemicalized foods and create blood sugar problems* that really do us in.

Ancient Civilizations And Low Fat Diets

Let's go back in time, with Drs. Mary and Michael Eades, in their book, *Protein Power*. The Eades start with the fact that "for 700,000 years humans ate a diet of mainly meat, fat, nuts

and berries. Eight thousand years ago we learned to farm, and as our consumption of grain increased, our health declined. Genetic evolutionary changes take a minimum of 1,000 generations – or *another* 8,000 to 10,000 years to adapt." [65]

In fact, the Drs. Eades note that anthropologists can tell whether the skull they are examining was that of a hunter-gatherer (protein eater) or a farmer (mainly carbohydrate eater). The well-formed, strong bones and teeth belong to the tall hunters. The farmers have signs of stunted growth and tooth decay.

Since there is so much information available to us about the ancient Egyptians, through their records and their mummies, they are a good starting point for historical nutritional evaluation. We know that they ate the perfect low-fat diet: lots of whole grains, fresh fruits and vegetables, along with some fish and fowl, and hardly any fat.

So what do paleopathologists find when they examine these mummies? (Paleopathology, among other modern techniques, applies forensic science to the early remains of man) They can tell why the corpse died, its age, sex, health status, and numerous other things.

"When paleopathologists dissected the arteries of the Egyptian mummies, they did not find smooth, supple arterial walls but rather arteries choked with greasy, cholesterol-laden deposits that were often calcified, exhibiting an advanced state of arteriosclerotic disease. Many subjects had arteries that were scarred and thickened, indicating the presence of high blood pressure. Pathologists today find the same diseased changes when examining tissue from a victim of heart attack, stroke, diabetes, or other disease found in conjunction with late-stage heart disease. In fact, it appears that cardiovascular disease was as prevalent in ancient Egypt as it is in America today." [66]

What's Happening Here?

Since humans were hunter-gatherers for such a long period, our metabolisms were designed to cope with food supplies that were unpredictable. What enabled us to store food for the lean times was *insulin.*

"Unfortunately, a diet heavy in carbohydrates also sends our insulin levels soaring, and our body interprets this as a need to store calories, to make cholesterol, and to conserve water — all important to our survival way back then." [67]

We would constantly have to be hooked up to our energy source (food) in order to merely function, if it were not for insulin. Insulin stores fat in our bodies, and this fat acts like a built-in battery, which gets re-charged when we eat, and used for energy when we don't.

So, diet is the best way to control insulin. In fact, it is the *only* way. Consumption of large quantities of carbohydrates produces large quantities of insulin because carbohydrates are really composed of various sugar molecules, or glucose, bonded chemically. Once you have eaten a carbohydrate, even a *complex* carbohydrate, your body has digestive enzymes that break these chemical bonds and release the sugar molecules into the blood.

"Insulin springs into action when the blood sugar starts to climb too high, as it does after a carbohydrate meal. The elevated blood sugar triggers the pancreas to synthesize and release insulin into the bloodstream. This insulin first makes a pass through the liver, where it shuts down any sugar production that may still be going on, then travels on to the rest of the body, where it acts on sensors or receptors scattered across the surfaces of muscle and fat cells. These receptors, when activated by insulin, initiate a series of reactions that pump sugar (along with protein and fat) from the blood into the interior of the cells for use now or storage for later. Insulin stimulates the fat cells to take up fat and sugar from the blood and store it away as body fat, especially in

the middle of the body, within the abdomen, and around the vital organs." [68]

Which Way Is Your Metabolism Going?

Since nature over and over again works with complementary factors (witness the bacteria-fungus relationship in plants), it is no wonder that our bodies have two hormones, *insulin* and *glucagon*, to store and release energy. Insulin causes our metabolism to store excess food energy for later and keeps our blood sugar from getting too high. Glucagon allows our bodies to burn our stored fat for energy and keeps our blood sugar from getting too low.

These functions of storing or burning fat are active to some degree all the time. The question is, which energy pathway predominates? Are we mainly storing or mainly burning fat for energy? It is important to note that the fat in the bloodstream could come from these sources:

1. Fat consumed in the diet.
2. Fat made from excess carbohydrates and protein in the diet.
3. Fat liberated from storage in the fat cells.

So, our bodies can make plenty of fat from carbohydrate — low-fat cookies and potato chips included.

In fact, the number-one foods consumed by most Americans are white bread, rolls and crackers. Number two are doughnuts, cookies and cake. Number three are alcoholic beverages. (Statistics from a survey performed in 1983 by the National Center for Health Statistics, which no longer conducts this survey.)

Drs. Michael and Mary Dan Eades point out that *the combination of high carbohydrates with low proteins caused the greatest increase in insulin production — more than carbohydrates themselves.* This is interesting, especially in light of the food Americans love, like hamburgers and fries, pizza, macaroni and

cheese, eggs and hash browns, cereal and milk, etc. — *all pro-tein/carbohydrate combinations.* The Eades also note that dietary fat in and of itself cannot cause problems with cholesterol unless you eat carbohydrates with the fat.

Dieting Is Failing

In a brilliant and controversial essay on intelligence published in the winter 1969 issue of *Harvard Educational Review,* Arthur R. Jensen, a professor of psychology at the University of California, Berkeley, wrote: "In other fields, when bridges do not stand, when aircraft do not fly, when machines do not work, when treatments do not cure, despite all conscientious efforts on the part of many persons to make them do so, one begins to question the basic assumptions, principles, theories, and hypotheses that guide one's efforts. Most physicians, dieticians and nutritionists have been locked in the notorious clean and well-lit prison on a single idea for decades. These experts have been treating obesity with low-calorie, low-fat, high-complex-carbohydrate diets, then standing around wringing their hands, watching 95% of their patients regain their weight. Perhaps inevitably they blame the patient for the failure." [69]

Obviously, the low-fat, high-carbohydrate diet is out of step with people's biochemistry — in fact, it actually strengthens an enzyme called *lipoprotein lipase*, a fat storage enzyme. To switch to a high-protein, low-carbohydrate diet keeps insulin levels low, so the lipoprotein lipase is not getting any stimulation. Instead, *hormone-sensitive lipase*, which releases fat from the fat cells into the blood, is stimulated.

More Than Just Fat

High insulin levels are the major cause of obesity, but according to Drs. Eades and the many medical studies they quote, all of

the following are symptoms of elevated insulin levels:

1. High blood pressure
2. High blood cholesterol and triglyceride levels
3. Diabetes (adult-onset specifically)
4. Heart disease

High Blood Pressure

Excessive insulin causes high blood pressure by forcing the kidneys to retain sodium, resulting in fluid retention. Excessive insulin also increases the thickness of the arterial walls, making them less elastic and more narrow, which drives the blood pressure up. In a final way, insulin stimulates the adrenals to constrict the blood vessels and increases the heart rate, thus raising blood pressure.

"Unfortunately, most doctors treat only the symptoms and often in a way that makes the real problem worse. If, for example, you go to your doctor and find that your cholesterol level and blood pressure are too high, we can just about guarantee that you will leave the office with instructions to go on a low-fat diet and to return to the office for a recheck in a month or so. If you follow this advice and go on the low-fat diet, what happens? By decreasing your fat intake you usually decrease your protein intake, because virtually all food that is protein-rich contains substantial amounts of fat. Meat, eggs, cheese and most dairy products — the best sources of complete dietary protein — are all taboo or severely restricted on a low-fat diet. With this protein and fat restriction, the only food component left in the diet is carbohydrate, which by default results in your eating a high-carbohydrate, low-protein diet — the very diet that maximizes insulin production. If you had hyperinsulinemia to begin with — and if you have elevated cholesterol and high blood pressure (and you can bet that you do) — increasing your body's produc-

tion of insulin isn't going to help. A month later, your doctor will probably find that your cholesterol has decreased slightly (because of the caloric restriction), but not enough to put it in the normal range, and that your blood pressure is about the same, maybe even a little higher. Now, when you leave the office, you'll go with a prescription for a high blood pressure medicine, a more stringent diet, and perhaps a prescription for a cholesterol-lowering medicine as well.

"You leave with your prescriptions, your sample medicines, your new diet instruction sheets and a nagging worry. You know that you followed the diet to the letter, so why didn't it work? And you wonder, 'Am I going to have to take these medicines for the rest of my life?' You comply with your doctor's orders and return at the appointed time for your follow-up visit. Your doctor finds that your blood pressure is down to normal and your cholesterol level has fallen into the normal range. You are relieved, and this time when you leave you're happy, your doctor is happy, and the drug companies are ecstatic: they have just signed you on as a new customer to the tune of between $50 and $300 per month for life.

"On the surface this story seems to have a happy ending, but does it really? While looking to the entire world like another triumph of modern medicine over disease, the treatment of your elevated cholesterol and high blood pressure is only a camouflage." [70]

WARNING: Drs. Michael and Mary Dan Eades found that a high protein/low carbohydrate diet was so effective in lowering blood pressure that their patents who were on medication to lower their blood pressure felt dizzy and faint within a few days and had to be taken off of their medication very quickly. So, do not attempt this diet if you are on medication to lower your blood pressure without being under the care of a physician.

Enter Cholesterol

At the beginning of the chapter in *Protein Power*, entitled "Cholesterol Madness," the Drs. Eades let you know that, with careful reading, "by the time you finish this chapter you will know more about cholesterol than 95 percent of the physicians in practice today." [71]

The problem is that cholesterol has become big business. "Whenever mass paranoia starts to brew, a legion rises up ready to exploit it. The food processing industry and their advertisers now emblazon the containers of edibles as diverse as soft drinks and cornflakes with the superfluous statement 'Contains no cholesterol.' Cholesterol angst is not lost on the various governmental and private research funding bodies responsible for underwriting all kinds of medical research. These groups disburse hundreds of millions of dollars to eager research labs throughout the world, allowing them to pursue the secrets of cholesterol in ever-more intricate studies." [72]

Cholesterol, as the Drs. Eades point out, is essential for life. Only 7% of the body's cholesterol is found in the blood. "The bulk of the cholesterol in your body, the other 93%, is located in every cell of the body, where its unique waxy, soapy consistency provides the cell membranes with their structural integrity and regulates the flow of nutrients into, and waste products out of, the cells." [73] Some cholesterol comes from food, but 80% is produced by the body itself, mostly by the liver.

Cholesterol is the building block for hormones and the major component of liver bile, and your brain and nerves need cholesterol for normal electrical signal transmission.

The number one point to remember is that the cholesterol levels are regulated *inside* the cell. When the supply runs low, the cell can either make more cholesterol or send LDL (low density lipoprotein) receptors (messengers) to the surface and snatch the next circulating LDL particle out of the blood.

LDL is sometimes seen as the villain in the cholesterol drama. And it can be if there is too much of it. But the truth is, there is again a natural relationship between LDL and HDL (high density lipoprotein). LDL carries cholesterol to the tissues for deposition and HDL gathers cholesterol from these tissues and carries it back to the liver to be disposed of. The flow one way or the other is what medical researchers have used to quantify risk for heart disease.

Insulin cranks up the cells' cholesterol-manufacturing ability so the cells don't need to snatch any from the bloodstream, and LDL levels rise. Clearly, the more LDL receptors we have pulling cholesterol from the blood, the better.

The artery-clogging damage that occurs with elevated insulin levels is analogous to "having a big thermostat that controls it into a small, hot, airtight closet. The cooling machinery could be cranking out throughout the house, but the thermostat in the closet would never know. As far as it knows, the air is hot and needs cooling, so it calls for more cold air; and in spite of the icicles forming on it, the air conditioner keeps huffing and struggling along to pump cold air out." [74]

By eating a diet that reduces insulin levels, "you reduce the signal telling the cells to make cholesterol; they *must* harvest it from the blood to have enough, and your blood cholesterol levels — especially the "bad" LDL — fall rapidly. Even while eating a diet that contains red meat, egg yolk, cheese, butter and cream, as long as you control your insulin output, your cholesterol will remain in the healthy 180-200 mg/dl range." [75]

Diabetes

As mentioned earlier, the United Nations and the World Health Organization, alarmed by mounting deaths due to cardiovascular disease and diabetes, issued a report in 2004 that predicted the number of cases of Type 2 diabetes, which is acquired, not inher-

ited, will soar from 117 million to 370 million by 2030. What causes diabetes?

In the case of Type 2 or Adult Onset Diabetes, a stage called "insulin resistance" or "impaired glucose tolerance" is first to appear. Starting in childhood, studies done in the United States have shown that many children from ages five on consume approximately one cup (200 grams) of sugar a day. If you included the starchy carbohydrates they consume, that figure would double. (Remember, *any* carbohydrate is metabolized exactly like sugar.)

After 30 or 40 years of this excess, the metabolic gears start to slip and middle age spread sets in. The person may even be eating less, but he/she is gaining weight. The insulin sensors in the tissues become more and more sluggish, and the pancreatic beta cells start working overtime to make more and more insulin to bring the blood sugar back into the normal range. At this point, if the blood glucose exceeds a certain threshold, typically 140 mg/dl, it will then be at such a high concentration in the blood that it destroys the beta cells.

This increase in blood sugar, in addition to going through the stage of insulin resistance to diabetes, has emotional components as well as physical. The "enriched" grains that most people consume cause vitamin depletion, especially the B complex. Some of the symptoms of B Complex Deficiency Syndrome, as it is called, are fatigue, nervousness, depression and forgetfulness.

Thomas Smith, author of *Insulin: Our Silent Killer*, has pointed out the following truth in the July-August edition of the *Nexus New Times* magazine: "For 40 years, medical research has consistently shown with increasing clarity that diabetes is a degenerative disease directly caused by an engineered food supply that is focused on profit instead of health."

The important thing to remember is that diet is the only method available to treat excess insulin. A high-protein, low-carbohydrate diet can reduce insulin levels in a matter of days and reduce blood

pressure and cholesterol or triglyceride levels. In a period of months, it can result in a steady loss of excess stored body fat. "Even though the regimen works rapidly to return insulin sensitivity to normal in most people, it works only as long as you follow it. It doesn't return you to your childhood levels of imperviousness to carbohydrate assault. You must continue to follow the guidelines to maintain the changes; a return to your former eating habits will return you to your former problems." [76]

Heart Disease

In the case of heart disease, problems arise when the flow of blood to any area of the heart is reduced significantly, or is cut off completely. Apparently the heart could pump on forever with adequate supplies of oxygen-rich blood.

When a person has a heart attack, it is usually brought on by a blockage of a coronary artery created by the build-up of plaque.

"Plaque forms over a long period of time, progressing in a stepwise fashion, starting with the infiltration of cholesterol into the lining of the artery and proceeding to the development of the mature lesion." [77]

The five steps in the plaque-forming process are:

1. Cholesterol in the LDL form makes its way into the arterial lining.
2. The trapped cholesterol becomes chemically altered.
3. Foam cells form. These are scavenger cells that eat the altered LDL and bloat up.
4. Fatty streaks form as there are more and more foam cells.
5. These fatty streaks collect to form plaque.

"*Insulin*, by its action on the cholesterol synthesis pathway located within the cells, helps to create and sustain excess amounts of LDL in blood ... and also increases the proliferation of smooth

muscle cells in the artery and their migration into the area of plaque formation." [78]

In the 1960s, Dr. Anatolio Cruz conducted an eight-month study on insulin by using dogs. Every day, insulin was injected into the large artery of one of the dog's legs. The other leg was injected with sterile saline. At the end of the eight-month period, the arteries injected with insulin had a pronounced accumulation of cholesterol and were already thickening. The leg injected with saline had no change. Imagine what years and years of excess insulin in the bloodstream can do.

Don't Forget The Eicosanoids

I have mainly used Drs. Michael and Mary Dan Eades' book to illustrate the importance of a high-protein, low-carbohydrate diet. But, *Dr. Atkins' New Dietary Revolution* and Dr. Barry Sears' *The Zone*, both expound the same dietary principles.

It is Dr. Sears who brought eicosanoids into the public arena. He even describes *optimal health* as the dynamic balance between the various eicosanoids.

"You can view eicosanoids as the biological glue that holds together the human body. In that regard they are the most powerful agents known to man, yet they are totally controlled by diet." [79]

Again, our body works as a balance of opposing forces. There are almost 100 powerful eicosanoids in the body. They control whether or not your blood vessels contract or dilate, whether or not you suffer from allergies, sleep well or poorly, whether or not you form tumors, and on and on. In fact, most cardiac drugs are eicosanoids inhibitors.

So, there are "good" and "bad" eicosanoids, and they are all produced from the dietary fat, *linoleic acid*, which is present in practically all foods. Essential fatty acids are the building blocks of eicosanoids, but linoleic acid is the only true essential fat from which all other fats can be made.

The Drs. Eades point out that foods have an influence on the eicosanoid factor at two different points:

1. Where linoleic acid enters the system. Since linoleic acid is found in nearly all foods, a person should have plenty available.
2. Where the critical gatekeeper enzyme delta 6 desaturase shifts the production to good or bad eicosanoids. Dietary protein is the only factor that speeds up this gatekeeper. The factors that slow it down are:

    (a) Aging
    (b) Stress
    (c) Disease
    (d) Trans-fatty acids, such as margarine and the partially-hydrogenated oils found in thousands of commercial foods "cause health damage because they inhibit the formation of the good eicosanoids." [80]
    (e) High-carbohydrate, low-protein diets stimulate excess insulin, which sends the production of bad eicosanoids soaring.

Obviously, there is not too much we can do about aging. Our fast-paced American way of life makes stress a common factor in almost everyone's life; no matter how hard we try, we can still get the occasional cold or flu.

Since aging, stress, and disease are pretty much beyond our control, we are left with the remaining three factors, all dietary. By exercising control and not consuming trans-fatty acids, adding good oils to our diets, and switching to a high protein, low-carbohydrate diet, we can do a lot to produce good eicosanoids and experience good health.

A Doctor's View

From the previous explanations of all of the havoc that excess insulin causes in our bodies, it is no wonder that more and more medical doctors are questioning the very principles on which our health system is based.

Dr. Atkins, in his *Health Revelations*. (Vol. IV, No. 4, May 1996), talks about the rigid orthodoxy of *Cecil's Textbook of Medicine*, which is the book that gets doctors through medical school. Atkins says that: *"Cecil's* teems with ... misinformation ... the book's common denominator is preservation of an outdated status quo, which can be summed up this way: 'Make sure non-pharmacological treatments fail, then prescribe drugs.' That rigid teaching is a miseducation and an unconscionable disservice to patients. A doctor who passed the boards because he or she knew everything in *Cecil's Textbook of Medicine* would have no value at the Atkins' Center. Treatment by textbook has no place in your health, either."* [81]

When Dr. Atkins' diet first came out, many considered him a rogue, some even calling him an "idiot." Today, Dr. Atkins' dietary principles of a low-carbohydrate, high protein, high fat diet are getting acknowledgement from all quarters of the medical community.

The growing frustration with standard medical views is also illustrated in the following:

"Robert D. Willix, Jr., M.D., was a hard-charging medical doctor who had developed the only open-heart surgery program in the state of South Dakota. He performed about 2,000 coronary bypass operations and finally realized he was not helping people. He has not picked up a scalpel since 1981; but, as he explains, 'I used to look at things the same way as the medical establishment. Basically, their view is that the body is a sort of machine you fix when it breaks down. I shucked off this dangerous, mistaken point of view and learned how human beings really work. Over the

past 40 years, evidence has been piling up that the way the body works is totally different from what the medical profession thinks'. Nevertheless, the medical way of thinking still prevails." [82]

It is important to note that Drs. Atkins, Eades, Sears, Willix, and others were the modern pioneers of this information. (The earlier works of Dr. Melvin Page, who pursued a low-carbohy-drate/high-protein diet rich in green leafy vegetables, was the real basis for these modern pioneers. His book, *Health vs. Disease*, is available at www.ifnh.org) It is also important to note that this information has often not yet "trickled down" to patients' visits with their family doctor, and they still may be getting the archaic and deadly low-fat message.

4/Our Health

"Nature has been making normal birds, butterflies, and animals for millions of years. If wild animals can do it why cannot we? Is it because they, by their instinct, select the right foods and do not meddle with Nature's foods by changing them?"

— Dr. Weston Price
Nutrition and Physical Degeneration

What is health? Sadly, we are not quite sure of what good health is anymore.

The World Health Organization (WHO) defines health as a "state of complete physical, mental, and social well-being and not merely the absence of disease or infirmity." [83]

Dr. Francis Pottenger (whose cat study is examined on my website, www.theperfectcrime.com), defined health as the result of an optimal diet, "one which provides man with the nutrients essential to regenerate his body cells; to enable him to mature regularly as determined by his normal [bone], physical, and mental characteristics; to resist disease; to reproduce his kind [in succeeding generations]; and to enable him to produce a livelihood for his family." [84]

We now have a couple of good definitions of what good health is. But to know how very few people actually have good health, we need to be able to open up our eyes and start looking around. What is poor health? Every day one sees people with pasty, sallow complexions, either yellow, gray, or sometimes even white. That they have poor blood quality or that something else is wrong is not even considered.

There is hardly a grocery store, fast food chain, or office you can enter without seeing someone with his/her wrists immobilized

in a brace for carpal-tunnel syndrome. We blame repetitive work for this; never does it occur to us that human ligaments are weakened by insufficient protein, vitamin C complex, and trace minerals.

Babies are born with all kinds of abnormalities, and we just figure that, statistically, this is the way it is. Many people are obese; yet, we never look at all of the carbohydrates they consume. (Nibbling on a low-fat cookie is even encouraged.) The consumption of sodas, pizza, and other fast food is rampant in our schools, and the numbers of obese children is skyrocketing. Other health problems, like varicose veins, easy bruising, bleeding gums, stretch-marks, popping or cracking of the joints, and slipped discs are just accepted as "normal wear and tear" on the body. No one would ever think that these are signs of *subclinical scurvy*, a C complex deficiency. Impaired wound-healing, hair loss, dry skin, and eczema are accepted as a part of our genetic makeup. However, these are all signs of a *vitamin F or fatty-acid deficiency*. (Remember, trans-fatty acids can *cause* vitamin F deficiencies).

We rationalize all this and more and keep on moving — but *tiredly*. Fatigue has gotten so common that we even have a syndrome devoted to it: *Chronic Fatigue Syndrome*.

Look In The Mirror

One of the most common nutritional deficiencies in America today is B Complex Deficiency (BCD). Some symptoms of BCD are:

Indigestion	Anxiety
Weakness and Fatigue	Depression
Dizziness	Mental Confusion
Forgetfulness	Fears
Uneasiness	Hostility
Rage	Craving for Sweets

The tendency to cry for no reason at all is one of the most com-

mon complaints. The second and most classical symptom of BCD is a constant feeling that something dreadful is about to happen. There are so many emotional components to nutritional deficiencies, especially a B vitamin deficiency. Yet, many people and their practitioners tend to think that something is wrong with them and don't recognize the deficiency. (It's *not* a Prozac™ deficiency — it's a B vitamin deficiency.)

Adelle Davis, in her book, *Let's Eat Right To Keep Fit*, points out that many changes take place in the tongue when the B vitamins are under supplied,.

"As the deficiencies of these vitamins become more severe, clumps of taste buds fuse and grow together, pulling apart from other clumps and thus forming grooves or fissures. The first groove usually forms down the center of the tongue. In a severe B-vitamin deficiency, the tongue may be so cut by grooves and fissures that it looks like a relief map of the Grand Canyon and the surrounding territory or a flank steak run through a tenderizing machine." [85] (Grab a mirror and look at your tongue.)

People who are in a "brain fog" are often deficient in B vitamins. Also, dim vision in the elderly, and swollen, red eyelids are symptoms of vitamin B deficiency. (vitamin B_2 specifically).

With some of these vitamin deficiencies as guidelines, you can see where many Americans are *starving* for different nutrients. Stop taking all of these deficiency signs for granted! Get to your health professional and get a proper evaluation and start on the road to health. Remember, wellness is the *only* health insurance.

Digestion vs. Indigestion

Well, by now we are all set to start eating more protein. But, we stop and think, one of the reasons many of us stopped eating meat was that it gave us heartburn. Also, sometimes after eating meat, we felt sluggish with the food just sitting in our stomachs.

Indigestion plagues almost everyone. Tagamet™ is the #1 selling drug in the world. Even vending machines carry Pepcid AC™ and

Tums™. "Epigastral reflux" is becoming a household word. So, indigestion is common; but, what exactly is *digestion*?

To digest food, stay immune from parasites, and avoid getting candida, you *must* have plenty of hydrochloric acid (HCl) in your stomach. This "arch-villain" in all the antacid commercials is *really a good guy.* In fact, your stomach is an acid machine.

When the stomach digests, it churns the food and mixes it with HCl, juices, pepsin, and enzymes. If there is no HCl, the food begins to rot and ferment. As it ferments, it then develops *abnormal acids* that are stinging and burning. Your stomach starts churning harder and harder, trying to digest the food in it, and sometimes some of these deviant acids, along with what little HCl remains, get backed up into the esophagus.

What you really need is more HCl, and to take an antacid at this point ensures that you have a mass of undigested food in your stomach. What doesn't get digested by your stomach then puts a burden on your liver and pancreas to get the job done, and they can't. Your body then begins to get toxic and full of poisons from this undigested matter.

Once again, Mother Nature designed the human body with a digestive assembly line to split open food molecules, break them down into vitamins, minerals, trace elements, fatty acids, amino acids and enzymes. Then your body eliminates what is not used through the bowel.

With an undigested food mass decaying and traveling through the 30 feet of the gastro-intestinal tract, all kinds of undesirable bacteria and viruses start scavenging this waste. Parasites, which could have been inadvertently swallowed and should have been destroyed by the HCl, are now finding a toxic environment in which to live. *Candida Albicans*, a fungus your body has in place to kill undesirable bacteria (remember the bacteria-fungus relationship in plants), starts to multiply to handle the ever larger volume of bacteria.

If this sounds disgusting, it is. The body is starting to break down through this continuous poisoning.

"If you have a concentration of bacteria living in some organ

of the body, you have a staph infection or strep in the throat, for instance, they are there because of unhealthy, devitalized tissue and unprocessed metabolic waste ... *disease is not the presence of something evil, but rather the lack of the presence of something essential.*"[86]

So, eating correctly is important, and digesting it is just as important! Standard Process makes an excellent HCl supplement, Zypan™, which also includes pancreatin and pepsin to help the stomach get the job done.

Summing Up

This book has been presented in an effort to educate you about natural food and soil, whole food supplements vs. synthetic vitamins, and the importance of protein and natural fats in the diet. It is an attempt to *go back to the basics of human health*, because it is in the basic diet of our forefathers that we are truly protected from all this craziness.

Good, whole food is the most important element in our lives. Food is the source of ALL nutrients required by the human body to perform its many biochemical processes. Without these required nutrients, the chemical processes are unable to complete themselves and run out of gas, so to speak. Since nutritional deficiencies are normally not life-threatening at first and take time to manifest themselves into serious health problems, many people ignore the early warning signs that their bodies are putting out, such as deteriorating joints, headaches, etc. In fact, all too often, these warning signs are dismissed as something that has to be lived with. "Oh, I'm just getting old," or "I have a high pain threshold," are phrases commonly heard.

As a result, existing deficiencies may eventually manifest themselves in varying degrees of illness through an abnormal pattern of symptoms. This depends on the person's state of health to begin with and what sort of foods he or she puts into his/her body day after day.

Going Back to the Basics is a return to foundational nutrition, which points to the root cause of ALL disease and symptoms as being a depleted diet and a sedentary lifestyle. These factors are then further impacted by the effect of sugar handling on vitamin and mineral metabolism. The long-term effects of inefficient sugar handling are poor digestion and impaired liver/gallbladder (biliary) function, resulting in a disruption of the endocrine system. This disruption stimulates multiple symptoms and problems. Examples of this can be seen in the numerous menopausal difficulties women are having today and the aggressive behavior of people that we hear so often about in the news.

But we now have other considerations to add to this picture: toxicity from heavy metals; the toll of decades of substandard foods being allowed to be produced; massive amounts of herbicides, pesticides, and fungicides being applied to growing foods; and, thousands of food additives that are allowed to be added to processed foods. All of these factors cause the breakdown of our normal immune systems. Hence, we now have auto-immune diseases we never heard of before.

Because this has happened over a span of time involving several generations, people have gradually come to accept marginal health as the norm, and so much of our modern living tends to desensitize people and hold them in a lethargic state. "Hollow food grown on empty soil keeps their bodies and minds dull, unproductive in manufacturing the chemical compounds of the brain and endocrine system. To once quote Surgeon General Parran, 'Many well-to-do Americans who can eat what they like are so badly fed as to be physically inferior and mentally dull.'

"Enfeebled as such, in this disconnected life, people actually don't want to know what is happening in reality, so they safely read about unreality in supermarket tabloids and popular magazines; which, no matter how outrageous the stories, require no response or action on their parts. They gulp their sugared soda pop and nibble on their hydrogenated chips, oblivious to the garbage and radiation that infiltrates their water, their air and their soil. Pathetically, their

biggest fear is 'losing it all.' Afraid of dying, the fear of truly living is greater.

"The feeling seems to be, 'There is only so much of the good life, not everyone can have it, and I am lucky to have my share. I don't know Mother Earth, but I'll rest my soul in the bosom of Mother General Mills, or Mother Exxon, or Mother Squibb, or Mother Del Monte, or Mother DuPont, or Mother Safeway.' Of course, loyalty to these 'mothers' is as deep as a paycheck or discount coupon." [87]

And then we wonder about the rising crime rate, problems with our children in school, and social problems of all kinds. It is an unhealthy world we live in. All we can do is start with ourselves. We need to get ourselves and our families healthy first, then our friends, and then work gradually out to our community and so on.

So, instead of running from one new "health discovery" to another and ignoring the way our forefathers ate, embrace it. Remember, over 100 years ago, people ate fresh whole foods including plenty of meat, butter and lard. *Go Back to the Basics!* It has been proven to work.

How Do We Find The Answers To Our Health Problems?

In the traditional medical role model of today, an exam would entail the doctor not touching you and barely taking the time to talk to you, then sending you off for some high-tech testing. Unfortunately, this kind of care has been stimulated by HMO business practices that look at the bottom line. With the influence of the drug companies, there is no interest in prevention. The more people that get sick, the slower they deteriorate, the more money there is to be made. If you really think about this, it becomes evident why so many people find themselves taking several prescription drugs a day. In fact, in some cases, people take in excess of a dozen prescription drugs daily. They start out with a drug to take care of one symptom. This drug usually creates side effects that require another drug — and on and on.

As a result, "every day more than 4,000 patients have adverse drug symptoms so serious that they need to be admitted to American

hospitals…In addition to the 1.5 million people a year who are admitted to the hospital *because* of adverse drug reactions, an additional three-quarters of a million people a year develop an adverse drug reaction *after* they are hospitalized." [88] (No wonder health insurance premiums are skyrocketing.)

Over 100,000 people a year die from adverse drug reactions, making them the 4th or 5th leading cause of death in America, depending on whose statistics you look at. The leading causes of death are heart disease, cancer, and strokes … and now adverse drug reactions.

All of us should have a copy of *Worst Pills Best Pills, A Consumer Guide to Avoiding Drug-Induced Death or Illness* (available at www.worstpills.org/buybooks). This book helps guide people through the deadly maze of prescription drug side effects and suffering.

An alternative health practitioner, on the other hand, is concerned about the patient's lifestyle and diet, which in most cases are the underlying cause of his or her health problems. This is a very different view from the traditional medical role model and requires some action on the part of the patient.

Take the example of JoAnn, who has been diagnosed with Chronic Fatigue Syndrome. Every morning, JoAnn got up and, after she left her house, stopped at Starbucks™ for a latte and a sweet roll. She also ate some fruit because she was trying to eat healthy. At 10:00am, she started to feel fatigued and would eat a candy bar and drink a diet soda from the vending machine at work. At lunch, she would eat a salad because she was trying to be healthy, and then she washed this down with another diet soda. At 3:00pm, she could hardly stay awake, so she would nibble on a cookie and drink some coffee. By the time she got home, she could hardly function. She was too tired to cook for her husband, so they grabbed something at a fast-food place.

If no one made her aware of the pitfalls of her lifestyle, she could easily be put on an anti-depressant to help her get through the day, but it still wouldn't do anything for her fatigue.

An alternative practitioner, looking at function, would use different tools to help her understand that she has a severe blood-sugar handling problem that is out of control, and has been out of control for years. Now she's starting to pay the price.

An alternative health practitioner might use the following tools. All of these tools look at function, not pathology, and many of the hands-on tests were used as part of the training process of doctors in medical schools until the 1950s. Although most of these tests could be run and interpreted with accuracy in five minutes, their use was discontinued in favor of machines and new technology, many times more expensive and time-consuming. This methodology lacks the personal contact the original standard tests offered to the all-important doctor/patient relationship. How soon we tend to forget quickness and simplicity in our misguided quest for the newest technological improvements.

1) **Symptom Survey Questionnaire**. This actually originated prior to the Cornell Questionnaire of the 1950s. Out of 194 symptoms, JoAnn has marked 103 of them. She has checked symptoms that indicate she is both hyper- and hypo-thyroid, both hyper- and hypo-adrenal, both hyper- and hypo-pituitary. What this indicates is a severe blood-sugar handling issue that is impacting her digestion, including pancreatic and gall bladder functions, and is congesting her liver.

2) **Nutritional Exam**. When JoAnn's Chapman Reflex Point was palpated for pancreatic function, it tested sensitive. When her digestive points were palpated, both showed a need for hydrochloric acid and pancreatin digestive enzyme support. Her gall bladder points were also sensitive.

3) **Acoustic CardioGraph™ (ACG) Machine**. Based on the original Endocardiograph machine invented by Dr. Royal Lee, this machine has a microphone that "listens" to the heartbeat and records the heart function graphically. The Endocardiograph was used extensively in doctors' offices and clinics throughout the United States during the 1940s, 1950s, and into the 1960s.

There has been some confusion between the ACG and the EKG. The ACG measures function based on acoustic signature of the heart sound, where the EKG measures trauma or damage to the heart with electrical current. (The ACG machine can be purchased through The Acoustic CardioGraph Company, (858) 488-2533, or visit their website, www.acg-co.com) In JoAnn's case, when the ACG was used, her severe blood sugar handling problem showed up as a vitamin B and vitamin E deficiency, a calcium deficiency, and a digestive and gall bladder issue. The graph also showed a major adrenal issue, which of course accounted for much of her fatigue. The body will beg, borrow, and steal from its reserves to keep the heart healthy. If the heart is not functioning optimally, then the body's reserves have been severely depleted, and, what has been eaten is not doing the job of maintaining optimum health.

4) **Reflex Analysis**. There are many reflex systems that have been developed over the last 70 years. Drs. DeJarnette, Rees, Barnett, Goodheart, and Versendaal have performed extensive research on their reflex systems. Many trials matching blood and urine work have proved the accuracy of reflex analysis in determining the cause of any condition. In JoAnn's case, a thorough exam of this type verified all of her digestive, gall bladder, and adrenal issues as well as vitamin deficiencies.

With all of this information in place relating to function as root cause, JoAnn is facing a dietary lifestyle change. The alternative health practitioner will recommend whole food supplements to support her digestive, gall bladder, adrenal, and B and E vitamin needs. But, unless she cuts her consumption of carbohydrates and sugar drastically, she will not know complete relief and be totally successful in her quest to feel better.

Action Steps To Function Optimally

Unfortunately, medical schools train doctors exclusively in allopathic medicine and trauma care. As a result, most doctors overlook prevention and health. At this point, it is obvious that people need certain basics. According to the Drs. Eades and others, they are as follows:

1. Plenty of protein, ranging from 60-90 grams/day for women and 80-110 grams/day for men. Be sure that, as much as you can, you eat antibiotic and hormone-free meat and eggs from chickens that are cage-free. Also, raw milk and raw milk products have the most live enzymes and vitamins. (Pasteurizing became necessary because of the sanitation problems in dairies years ago. Today, these raw milk dairies are inspected frequently and have to meet a much higher standard than the dairies where milk is pasteurized.)

2. Plenty of fresh vegetables (especially the green leafy ones) and a limited number of fruits. All of these should be eaten in their whole form, *not juiced* (Take a look at the amount of carbohydrates and sugars in juices. Also, take a look at all the fructose and high fructose corn syrup in juices and avoid them. Studies have shown that fructose by-passes your body's regulatory mechanisms — it by-passes insulin and a key regulatory phase in the ATP process, building up levels of lactate, uric acid, and triglycerides.). The carbohydrate content of vegetables and fruits should be no more than 60 grams a day. (Thirty grams a day are recommended to lose weight, so you will need to purchase a carbohydrate and protein gram counter.) Make sure that the produce purchased is "certified organic." Again, in California, this means that farmers cannot use chemical fertilizers or pesticides for the previous three years. The soil is built up through organic means. After three years, the produce grown on this land is tested for pesticide residue. If there is none, then the label "certified organic" can be put on the produce; and in most cases, this produce has from 90% to 250% more nutrients than

commercially grown produce. *If "certified organic" is not available, eat fresh produce anyway.* Just be sure to peel your fruit and throw out the outer leaves of leafy vegetables. (See my website, www.theperfectcrime.com, for a defining study on organic vs. commercial produce.)

3. Water. Drink a minimum of six to eight glasses a day. (Avoid tap water. Drink purified water instead).

4. Exercise. You can't be optimally healthy just sitting or lying down all day long. You can start with a Step-O-Meter, which will tell you just how active you are. Then you can start adding steps to get to your goal. If you want to start amping up your exercise at that point, Covert Bailey's *Fit or Fat* book is a great next step. He recommends 20 minutes at maximum heart rate three times a week to burn fat.

5. One to three teaspoons of raw olive oil, fish oil, or flax seed oil every day. And use butter, too.

6. Adequate amounts of all important vitamins and minerals taken daily in the form of whole food supplements, and whatever digestive enzymes you need. Remember, *supplements are the means of catching up for lost time nutritionally.* All of these should be determined by a health care professional.

I hope that the information in this book will set you firmly on the path to wellness.

Ode To A Shelf-Life

Ah, but to last longer on the shelf

It certainly has made an industry of wealth

To enrich, store and transport has been the goal

My body doesn't know the difference, I am told

If I could but last as long as thee

Oh, odorless oils, canned foods, cereal and candy.
— *Anonymous*

Appendix

Footnotes

1. Jensen, Dr. Bernard and Mark Anderson, *Empty Harvest,* p. 14.
2. *Ibid,* p. 5.
3. *Ibid,* p. 73.
4. von Liebig, Baron Justus, *The Natural Laws of Husbandry.*
5. Jensen, Dr. Bernard and Mark Anderson, *Empty Harvest,* p. 75.
6. Howard, Sir Albert, *An Agricultural Testament,* Oxford University Press.
7. Jensen, Dr. Bernard and Mark Anderson, *Empty Harvest,* p. 32.
8. *Ibid,* pp. 57-58.
9. *New Yorker* magazine, April 10, 2000, p. 58.
10. Jensen, Dr. Bernard and Mark Anderson, *Empty Harvest,* pp. 46-47.
11. *Ibid,* p. 8.
12. *Ibid,* p. 55.
13. *Ibid,* p. 7.
14. *Ibid,* p. 27.
15. *Ibid.*
16. *Ibid,* p. 97.
17. *Ibid,* p. 37.
18. Wiley, Dr. Harvey W., MD, *The History of a Crime Against the Pure Food Law,* p. 391.
19. *Ibid,* pp. 401-402.

20. *The Washington Post*, October 26, 1949.
21. Jensen, Dr. Bernard and Mark Anderson, *Empty Harvest,* p. 36.
22. *Ibid,* p. 38.
23. *Ibid.*
24. *Ibid.*
25. *Ibid,* p. 39.
26. *Ibid,* pp. 126-127.
27. West, Bruce, M.D., "Oils and Disease," *Health Alert,* Vol. II, issue 3, (March 1994), p. 4; Dorman, Thomas A., M.D., *Search for Health,* (November 1994), p. 100.
28. DeCava, Judith A., M.S., LNC, *The Real Truth About Vitamins and Antioxidants*, p. 134.
29. Stitt, Paul A., *Beating The Food Giants*, p. 53.
30. DeCava, Judith A., M.S., LNC, *The Real Truth About Vitamins and Antioxidants*, p. 140.
31. www.fluoridealert.org
32. *The Merck Manual of Medical Information*, p. 709.
33. DeCava, Judith A., M.S., LNC, *The Real Truth About Vitamins and Antioxidants*, p. 76.
34. *Ibid,* p. 37
35. *Ibid,* p. 38..
36. Cheraskin, AE. And W.M. Ringsdorf, Jr., *New Hope for Incurable Diseases* (Jericho: Exposition, 1971), pp. 83-85.
37. DeCava, Judith A., M.S., LNC, *The Real Truth About Vitamins and Antioxidants*, p. 37.
38. Carter, Dr. James P., M.D., Dr.P.H., *Racketeering in Medicine*, pp. 23-24, citing David Horrobin, M.D., *Journal of the American Medical Association,* March 1990), and Charles Harris, Pathologist, *Cult of Medical Science.*
39. Williams, Dr. Robert J., *Nutrition Against Disease*, pp. 4, 5, 11, 17.

40. Krause, Marie V., B.S., M.S., R.D., and Kathleen Mahan, M.S., R.D., *Food, Nutrition and Diet Therapy*, (Philadelphia: W.B. Saunders Company, 1979), pp. 148-149.

41. DeCava, Judith A., M.S., LNC, *The Real Truth About Vitamins and Antioxidants*, p. 51.

42. *Ibid,* p. 57.

43. *Ibid,* p. 59.

44. Lee, Dr. Royal, *Vitamin News*, Vol. 8, p. 135.

45. DeCava, Judith A., M.S., LNC, *The Real Truth About Vitamins and Antioxidants*, p. 54

46. *Ibid,* p. 117.

47. *Ibid,* p. 119.

48. *Ibid,* p. 163.

49. *Ibid,* p. 190.

50. Jensen, Dr. Bernard and Mark Anderson, *Empty Harvest*, p. 123.

51. DeCava, Judith A., M.S., LNC, *The Real Truth About Vitamins and Antioxidants*, p. 41.

52. *Ibid,* p. 64.

53. Toufexis, Anastasia, *Time Magazine,* (April 6, 1992), pp. 54-59.

54. DeCava, Judith A., M.S., LNC, *The Real Truth About Vitamins and Antioxidants*, p. 96.

55. *Ibid,* p. 70.

56. Challem, Jack, "Are You Overdoing Antioxidants?," *Natural Health*, Vol. 25, No. 3, (May/June 1995), pp. 56-57.

57. Jensen, Dr. Bernard and Mark Anderson, *Empty Harvest*, p. 25.

58. *Ibid,* p. 47.

59. *Ibid,* pp. 47-48.

60. Murray, Richard P., D.C., P.A., *Natural vs. Synthetic, Life vs. Death, Truth vs. The Lie*, 1995, p. 4.

61. *Ibid.*

62. *Ibid,* p. 5.
63. West, Bruce, M.D., *Health Alert*, Vol. 14, No. 3 (March 1997).
64. Rodale, J.I., *The Complete Book of Food and Nutrition*, cited in *Empty Harvest*, pp. 127-128.
65. Eades, Michael R., M.D. and Mary Dan Eades, M.D., *Protein Power*, p. 21.
66. *Ibid,* p. 15.
67. *Ibid,* p. 21.
68. *Ibid,* p. 32.
69. Jensen, Arthur R., Ph.D., *Harvard Educational Review,* (Winter 1969) cited in *Protein Power*, pp. 51-52.
70. Eades, Michael R., M.D. and Mary Dan Eades, M.D., *Protein Power,* pp. 40-41.
71. *Ibid,* p. 93.
72. *Ibid,* pp. 92-93.
73. *Ibid,* p. 94.
74. *Ibid,* p. 96.
75. *Ibid,* p. 114.
76. *Ibid,* p. 41.
77. *Ibid,* p. 64.
78. *Ibid,* p. 66.
79. Sears, Dr. Barry, *The Zone*, p. 32.
80. Eades, Michael R., M.D. and Mary Dan Eades, M.D., *Protein Power*, p. 80.
81. Atkins, Dr. Robert, *Health Revelations,* Vol. 4, No. 5, (May 1996).
82. Willix, Robert D., Jr., M.D., *Maximum Health,* (Baltimore: Agora, Inc, 1993), pp. 33-35, cited in *The Real Truth About Vitamins and Antioxidants*, p. 35.
83. Pottenger, Francis M., Jr., M.D. *Pottenger's Cats*, p. 93.
84. *Ibid.*
85. Davis, Adelle, M.S., *Let's Eat Right To Keep Fit*, p. 66.

86. Jensen, Dr. Bernard and Mark Anderson, *Empty Harvest*, p.113.
87. *Ibid,* pp. 153-154.
88. *Worst Pills Best Pills*, p. 9.

Suggested Reading

1. Nutrition and Physical Degeneration, Weston A. Price, D.D.S. (www.ifnh.org)
2. Empty Harvest, Dr. Bernard Jensen and Mark Anderson (www.ifnh.org)
3. The Real Truth About Vitamins and Antioxidants, Judith A. DeCava, M.S., LNC (www.ifnh.org)
4. Health vs. Disease, Melvyn Page, D.D.S. (www.ifnh.org)
5. Protein Power, Michael R. Eades, M.D. and Mary Dan Eades, M.D. (www.amazon.com)
6. Health Alert, a monthly newsletter by Dr. Bruce West, (831) 372-2103
7. www.saveteeth.org - fluoride information
8. Why Do I Need Whole Food Supplements?, Lorrie Medford, C.N. (www.ifnh.org)
9. Vitamin News, Dr. Royal Lee (www.ifnh.org)
10. Worst Pills Best Pills (www.worstpills.org/buybooks)
11. Pottenger's Cats, Dr. Francis Pottenger, Jr. (www.ifnh.org)
12. The Zone, Dr. Barry Sears (www.amazon.com)
13. The Facts About Fats, John Finnegan (www.amazon.com).

Index

- A -

abnormalities 72
absorption,
    calcium and magnesium 41
acid,
    acetic 41
    ascorbic 29,32,34,35, 36,
    42,43
    benzoic 18
    citric 25
    fluosilicic 27,28
    folic 53
    linoleic 66,67
    polyunsaturated fatty 42
    pyruvic 36
    uric 81
acids,
    abnormal 74
    amino 74
    essential fatty 66
    fatty 74
    trans-fatty 25, 67,72
    unsaturated fatty 26
Acoustic CardioGraph™ (ACG)
    20,79
activators 32,36
additives 16
additives, food 76
adrenals 60
Africa, East 5
AF Betafood™ 52

Agriculture, Dept. of (USDA) 4,18
AIDS 15
Albrecht, William 13
alum 18
American Diabetes Association 1
Anderson, Mark 16,20
anthropologists 56
antioxidants 32,36,42,44,53
    synthesized 43
    synthetic 43,44
anxiety 72
An Agricultural Testament 8
arbohydrate 58
arteriosclerosis 24
arthritis 23
artificially color 16
ascorbic acid 32,34,35,36,41,42,43
Atkins, Robert 55
Atkins' Center 68
ATP process 81

- B -

bacteria 74
bacteria, infectious 41
Bailey, Covert 82
balance, acid/alkaline 41
beets, organic 52
beriberi 40
beta-carotene 31,42,43
Betafood™ 52
beta-carotene 38

beverages, alcoholic 58
biochemistry 34,59
biotechnology 12
bleached 45
blood
       cholesterol 60
       glucose 64
       pressure 60,61,64
       sugar 55,57,64
       sugar handling 79,80
       vessels 60
boron 14
bowel 74
bread, white 26,58
bronchitis 41
buckwheat juice 38
Bureau of Chemistry 16
butter 63,82
B Complex Deficiency (BCD) 72

- C -

C, vitamin 29
caffeine 18
cancer 15,24,25,78
Candida Albicans 74
carbohydrate, complex 57
carbohydrates 55,57,58,64,65,72,
      80,81
      refined 23
carrot powder 38,53
Catalyn™ 51
Cataplex B™ 38,39
Cataplex E™ 52
Cecil's Textbook of Medicine 68
cellular combustion 44
Center for Disease Control 1
Center for Science in the Public
      Interest 23
cereal 59,83
certified organic 11,81,82
Chapman Reflex Point 79

cheese 63
chemical, man-made 16
chemically preserved 45
chemicals, synthetic 32,42
chemical fertilizer 11,16,81
children, obese 72
chlorophyll 24
cholesterol 57,60,61,62,63,65
chromium 14
Chronic Fatigue Syndrome 72,78
citric acid 25
co-enzyme 31,32,36
co-enzyme PQQ 53
co-enzyme Q-10 53
coal tar 30,32,34,54
cobalt 14
commerce, interstate 18
Complete Book of Food and Nutri-
      tion, The 54
complex,
      natural food 44
      nutritional 34
      vitamin 34,42
      vitamin B 37
      vitamin C 34,35,41,72
      whole B 41
      whole food 39,42,52
concentrates,
      food 34
      whole food 32
Consumer's Dictionary of Food
      Additives 30
Cornell University 11
cream 63
Cruz, Anatolio 66

- D -

d-Alpha succinate 38
d-Alpha tocopherol 42,53
Davis, Adelle 73
DeCava, Judith 31,37,43

defibered 16
deficiencies,
    dietary 19
    nutritional 45,75
    vitamin 73
    vitamin F 72
    B vitamin 73
deficiency,
    B Complex 72
    calcium 80
    C complex 72
    fatty-acid 72
    thiamin (B_1) 39
    trace mineral 45
    vitamin B 73
    vitamin C 36
    vitamin E 40,80
Deforestation 4
degeneration,
    kidney 24
    liver 24
delta 6 desaturase 67
depression 27,64
deteriorating joints 75
diabetes 3,15,23,24,56,60,63,64
    Adult Onset 64
diacetyl 25
diathesis, severe hemorrhagic 29
diet 58,78
    depleted 76
    high complex carbohydrate 59
    high-protein, low-carbohy-drate 61,64,66,67
    low-carbohydrate 59
    low-carbohydrate/high-pro-tein 69
    low-fat 60
    low-protein 60
    high-carbohydrate, low-pro-tein 67

difficulties, menopausal 76
digestion 52,76,79
diglycerides 25
discs, slipped 72
disease 76
    Alzheimer's 24
    arteriosclerotic 56
    auto-immune 76
    cardiovascular 24,56
    degenerative 64
    heart 56,60,63,65,78
    thyroid 27
    degenerative 19,23
    functional 19
    infectious 19
dl-Alpha tocopherol 38
Dr. Atkins' New Dietary Revolution 66
drugs, prescription 77
dry skin 72

- E -

Eades, Michael and Mary Dan 55,58,61,66
eater,
    carbohydrate 56
    protein 56
eczema 72
eggs 59,63, 81
eicosanoids 66,67
EKG 80
Empty Harvest 16,22,41
Endocardiograph 79
endocrine system 76
enriched 64
Environmental Protection Agency (EPA) 4,27
enzyme 50,51,59,67
    pancreatin digestive 79
enzymes 14,26,32,36,53,74,81,82
    digestive 57

esophagus 74
Exam, Nutritional 79
eyelids, swollen, red 73

- F -

factor, anti-paralysis 38
Facts About Fats, The 25
farmer 56
fast food 71,72
fat 57,58,59
fatigue 36,44,64,80
fats 24,55
      high blood 52
      natural 75
Fat Burning Diet ix
FDA 16,18,20,22,23,25,28,29,30,3
      1,35,39,51
fertilizer,
      chemical 8
      phosphate 27
Finnegan, John 25
Fit or Fat 82
flour,
      bleached 18
      enriched 30
fluid retention 60
fluoride,
      calcium 26
      sodium 26
Folic acid 53
Folk Medicine 41
food,
      devitalized 19,23
      processed 76
      unadulterated 23
foods,
      adulterated 49
      canned 83
      chemicalized 55
      commercial 67
      fresh whole 77
foods of commerce 49
*Food & Life: The United States
      Department of Agriculture
      Yearbook for 1939* 19
food additives 76
Food and Drug Administration
      (FDA) 16
food concentrates 34
forgetfulness 64
fortified, synthetically 16
free radical 42,43
fructose 81
function,
      gall bladder 52,79
      impaired liver/gallbladder 76
      pancreatic 41,79
fungicides 4,11,16,76
Funk & Wagnall 29
Future of Food, The 12

- G -

gall bladder 52,79,80
gardening, organic 49
gastro-intestinal tract 74
General Mills 23
germ, organic wheat 52
Glickman, Dan 5
glucagon 58
glucose 57
*Going Back to the Basics of Human
      Health* viii
gram counter 81
gums, bleeding 72

- H -

H.J. Heinz Nutrition Chart 9
hair loss 27,72
Hamaker, John D. 15
hamburgers 58

handling, blood-sugar 79
Harman, Denham 43
Harvard Educational Review 59
Harvard School of Public Health 26
HDL (high density lipoprotein) 63
headaches 27,75
Health Alert 52
Health Revelations 68
Health vs. Disease 69
heartburn 73
heart
       attack 56,65
       disease 3,15
       problem 52
heavy metals 76
Hensel, Julius 8,51
herbicides 76
high potency 39
homogenized 16,31,45
hormone-sensitive lipase 59
Howard, Albert 8
hunter-gatherer 56,57
hydrochloric acid (HCl) 74,79
hydrogenated 16
hyperinsulinemia 60
hypertension 3
hypothyroidism 27

- I -

imbalance, bio-chemical 34
immune system 27,43
impaired glucose tolerance 64
insulin 57,58,59,60,63,64,66,67,68
Insulin: Our Silent Killer 64
International Foundation for Nutri-
      tion and Health iii,22,52
isopropyl 25

- J -

Jarvis, D. C. 41
Jensen, Arthur R. 59

Jensen, Bernard 16,20,41
*Journal of the American Medical
      Association* 27
*Journal of Toxicology and Environ-
      mental Health* 28
juices, vegetable 52

- K -

kidneys 36

- L -

lactate 81
LDL (low density lipoprotein)
      62,65
lecithin 24
Lee, Royal 13,19,37,45,50,53,79
Lee Foundation iii
Lee Foundation for Nutritional
      Research 22
Let's Eat Right To Keep Fit 73
Liebig, Baron Justus von 8
lifestyle 78
      dietary 80
      sedentary 76
linoleic acid 66,67
lipoprotein lipase 59
liver 34,36,38,40,53,57,62,79
liver, organic 52
liver bile 62

- M -

macaroni and cheese 58
malnutrition 23
      Cellular 32,35
Malone, Dorothy 22
margarine 25
marketing, multi-level 30
Materia Medica 40
meat, hormone-free 81
Merck Manual 1

metabolism,
    calcium 26
    mineral 76
method,
    bioassay 35
    scientific 34
methyl isocyanate 11
micronutrient 51
mineral 23,74,82
monoglycerides 25
Montaigne 1
Morgan, Agnes Fay 19
Mother Jones 12
Mother Nature 4,41,53,74
multiple sclerosis 24
mummies, Egyptian 56
muscular weakness 44
mycorrhiza 13

- N -

NASA 20
National Center for Health Statistics
    58
native americans 4
natural food complexes 44
Nelson, Elmer M. 19
nervousness 64
New Diet Revolution ix
New Yorker 12
New York Times Magazine 55
Nexus New Times 64
Niacin 39
nutrient, 42
    organic 32
    food-sourced 31
Nutrient Testing Laboratory 9
nutrition 30
Nutritional Action 23
Nutritional Exam 79
*Nutrition and Physical Degenera-
    tion* 49,71

- O -

obesity 15,59
OCEANA 11
oil,
    fish 82
    flax seed 53,82
    irradiated 54
    polyunsaturated 25
    raw olive 82
    wheat germ 34
oils 24,26
    fish 26
    flax seed 26
    fresh-pressed organic 52
    good 67
    natural 26
    odorless 83
    partially-hydrogenated 26,67
optimal health 66
organic 30
    farming 15
oxidation 42,43,44

- P -

Page, Melvin 23,69
paleopathologists 56
paleopathology 56
pancreas 57
pancreatic function 41
parasites 74
Parran, Surgeon General 76
pasteurized 16,45,81
pathologists 56
pathology 79
pathway, cholesterol synthesis 65
peavine plant 38
Pepcid AC™ 73
Perfect Crime, The 11,12,32,71,82
pesticides 4,11,16,31,76,81

pH
    alkaline 41
    balance 41
phyto-chemicals 53
Pimental, David 11
pizza 58,72
plaque 65
pneumonia 41
pollutants 4
poor memory 27
Pottenger, Francis 19,23,71
practices, HMO business 77
practitioner, alternative health 78
preservatives 16
pressure, high blood 56
Price, Weston 19,23,49,71
processes, biochemical 75
Product Bulletin 51
protein 55,57,58,73,75,81
    dietary 67
    insufficient 72
Protein Power 55,62
Prozac™ 73
pulmonary problems 41
Pure Food and Drug Law 16
pycnogenols 38,53

- Q -

Questionnaire,
    Cornell 79
    Symptom Survey 79

- R -

Real Truth About Vitamins and Anti-
    oxidants, The 31
raw milk products 81
RDA 35
reaction, adverse drug 78
Red Cross 39
red meat 63
Reflex Analysis 80

relationship, bacteria-fungus 58,74
research, vitamin 31
retinal palmitate 38
rice 40
Robb, Jay ix
Rodale, J. I. 54

- S -

saccharin 18
salt 16
scientific studies 35
scurvy 35
scurvy, subclinical 72
Sears, Barry 66
selective absorption 34
selenium 14,31,53
sensitivity, insulin 65
side effects 78
Simkovich, V.G. 15
Smith, Thomas 64
soda pop 72,76
sodium 60
sodium benzoate 25
soft drink 18
soybean 12
Standard Process 39,50,51,52,53
Starbucks™ 78
stearyl citrates 25
Step-O-Meter 82
sterilized 45
stroke 56,78
substances, isolated 42
sugar 16,23,57,80,81
    elevated blood 57
    handling 76
sulfites 18
sulfurous acid 18
supplement,
    organic 31
    whole food 51
    nutritional 32,42

vitamin 45
supplements, whole food 52,53, 80,82
Supreme Court 18
Sure, Barnett 49
Survival of Civilization, The 15
symptoms 76
Symptom Survey Questionnaire 79
syndrome,
    B Complex Deficiency 64
    carpal-tunnel 72
    Chronic Fatigue 72,78
synthetic vitamins 49,55
syrup, high fructose corn 81
system,
    endocrine 26,76
    immune 26,76
system, parasympathetic nervous 41
Szent-Gyorgi, Albert von 29

T

Tagamet™ 73
Taubes, Gary 55
theobromine 18
theory, free radical 43
therapeutic 29,51
Therapeutic Food Company 51
Therapeutic Food Manual 51
thiamine (B_1) 36,39,40
    HCL 39,54
    mononitrate 54,58
thyroid 27
tissue, devitalized 75
tocopherols 40
tooth decay 23,56
toxicity 76
toxic overdose 34
toxins 36
trace elements 32,74
trace mineral 14,31,53,72

trans-fats 25,26
triglyceride 60,65,81
Tums™ 74

U

U.S. vs. Lexington Mill and Elevator Company 18
uneasiness 72
United Nations 1,63
University of
    California, Berkeley 59
    Florida 50
    Missouri 13
uric acid 81
USDA 5

V

varicose veins 72
vegetables,
    fresh 81
    leafy 45
vinegar, apple cider 41
virus 74
vision, dim 73
vital organs 58
vitamin 23,76
    natural 31
vitamins 45,74,81,82
    artificial 23
    crystalline-pure 34,36
    synthetic 16,30,32,34,36,37, 44,45,49
vitamin
    A 31,38
    B 80
    B_1 39
    B_3 38
    B_4 38
    B_6 39
    B_{12} 14,53,54
    C 3,12,31,32,34,36,38,41,

42,43
D 38,54
E 24,31,38,40,42,43,53,80
F 72
fractions 31
Vitamin News 37,51

W

waste, unprocessed metabolic 75
water, purified 82
Webster's Dictionary 30,44
weight gain 27
wellness 73,82
West, Bruce 52
wheat germ 18
white blood cell 41
whole foods 15,24,29,40,75
whole food complex 35
Wiley, Harvey W. 16
Williams, Roger 19
Willix, Jr. Robert D. 68
Winter, Ruth 30
World Health Organization (WHO)
      1,63,71
Worst Pills Best Pills 78
wound-healing, Impaired 72
www.acg-co.com 80
www.ifnh.org 19,22,69
www.worstpills.org/buybooks 78

Y

yeast 34,40
yeast, high-selenium 52

Z

zinc 31
Zone, The 66
Zyclan B™ 11
Zypan™ 22,75